Outpatient Ultrasound-Guided Musculoskeletal Techniques

Editor

EVAN PECK

PHYSICAL MEDICINE AND REHABILITATION CLINICS OF NORTH AMERICA

www.pmr.theclinics.com

Consulting Editor
SANTOS F. MARTINEZ

August 2016 • Volume 27 • Number 3

ELSEVIER

1600 John F. Kennedy Boulevard ● Suite 1800 ● Philadelphia, Pennsylvania, 19103-2899

http://www.theclinics.com

**PHYSICAL MEDICINE AND REHABILITATION CLINICS OF NORTH AMERICA Volume 27, Number 3
August 2016 ISSN 1047-9651, ISBN 978-0-323-45985-3**

Editor: Jennifer Flynn-Briggs
Developmental Editor: Donald Mumford

Reprints. For copies of 100 or more of articles in this publication, please contact the Commercial Reprints Department, Elsevier Inc., 360 Park Avenue South, New York, NY 10010-1710. Tel.: 212-633-3874; Fax: 212-633-3820; E-mail: reprints@elsevier.com.

Physical Medicine and Rehabilitation Clinics of North America (ISSN 1047-9651) is published quarterly by Elsevier Inc., 360 Park Avenue South, New York, NY 10010-1710. Months of issue are February, May, August, and November. Business and Editorial Offices: 1600 John F. Kennedy Blvd., Suite 1800, Philadelphia, PA 19103-2899. Customer Service Office: 3251 Riverport Lane, Maryland Heights, MO 63043. Periodicals postage paid at New York, NY and additional mailing offices. Subscription price per year is $280.00 (US individuals), $538.00 (US institutions), $100.00 (US students), $335.00 (Canadian individuals), $709.00 (Canadian institutions), $210.00 (Canadian students), $415.00 (foreign individuals), $709.00 (foreign institutions), and $210.00 (foreign students). Foreign air speed delivery is included in all *Clinics* subscription prices. All prices are subject to change without notice. **POSTMASTER:** Send address changes to *Physical Medicine and Rehabilitation Clinics of North America*, Customer Service Office: Elsevier Health Sciences Division, Subscription Customer Service, 3251 Riverport Lane, Maryland Heights, MO 63043. **Customer Service: 1-800-654-2452 (US). From outside of the United States, call 314-447-8871. Fax: 314-447-8029. E-mail: JournalsCustomer Service-usa@elsevier.com (for print support); JournalsOnlineSupport-usa@elsevier.com (for online support).**

Physical Medicine and Rehabilitation Clinics of North America is indexed in *Excerpta Medica, MEDLINE/PubMed (Index Medicus), Cinahl,* and *Cumulative Index to Nursing and Allied Health Literature.*

Contributors

CONSULTING EDITOR

SANTOS F. MARTINEZ, MD, MS
Diplomate of the American Academy of Physical Medicine and Rehabilitation, Certificate of Added Qualification Sports Medicine, Campbell Clinic, Assistant Professor, Department of Orthopaedics, University of Tennessee, Memphis, Tennessee

EDITOR

EVAN PECK, MD
Staff Physician, Section of Sports Health, Department of Orthopaedic Surgery, Cleveland Clinic Florida, West Palm Beach, Florida; Affiliate Assistant Professor of Biomedical Science, Charles E. Schmidt College of Medicine, Florida Atlantic University, Boca Raton, Florida

AUTHORS

DENA ABDELSHAHED, MD
Department of Physical Medicine and Rehabilitation, Rutgers University-New Jersey Medical School, Newark, New Jersey

SEAN W. COLIO, MD
Instructor of Sports Medicine, Department of Physical Medicine and Rehabilitation, Swedish Spine, Sports, and Musculoskeletal Center, Swedish Medical Group, Seattle, Washington

MEDERIC M. HALL, MD
Associate Professor, Departments of Orthopedics and Rehabilitation, Radiology, and Family Medicine, University of Iowa Sports Medicine Center, Iowa City, Iowa

P. TROY HENNING, DO
Assistant Professor, Department of Physical Medicine and Rehabilitation, University of Michigan, Ann Arbor, Michigan

MARK-FRIEDRICH B. HURDLE, MD
Consultant; Assistant Professor, Departments of Physical Medicine and Rehabilitation and Pain Medicine, Mayo Clinic, Jacksonville, Florida

PRATHAP JAYARAM, MD
Department of Physical Medicine and Rehabilitation, Baylor College of Medicine, Houston, Texas

ELENA JELSING, MD
Assistant Professor, Department of Physical Medicine and Rehabilitation, Mayo Clinic College of Medicine, Mayo Clinic Sports Medicine Center, Minneapolis, Minnesota

DANIEL R. LUEDERS, MD
Sports Medicine Fellow, Department of Physical Medicine and Rehabilitation, Mayo Clinic
Sports Medicine Center, Mayo Clinic, Rochester, Minnesota

GERARD MALANGA, MD
Department of Physical Medicine and Rehabilitation, Rutgers University-New Jersey
Medical School, Newark, New Jersey; New Jersey Regenerative Institute, Cedar Knolls,
New Jersey

KEN MAUTNER, MD
Associate Professor, Departments of Orthopaedic Surgery and Physical Medicine and
Rehabilitation, Emory University, Atlanta, Georgia

KENTARO ONISHI, DO
Assistant Professor, Department of Physical Medicine and Rehabilitation, University of
Pittsburgh Medical Center, Pittsburgh, Pennsylvania

JEFFREY M. PAYNE, MD
Instructor, Physical Medicine and Rehabilitation, Mayo Clinic Health System, Faribault,
Minnesota

EVAN PECK, MD
Staff Physician, Section of Sports Health, Department of Orthopaedic Surgery, Cleveland
Clinic Florida, West Palm Beach, Florida; Affiliate Assistant Professor of Biomedical
Science, Charles E. Schmidt College of Medicine, Florida Atlantic University, Boca Raton,
Florida

ADAM M. POURCHO, DO
Instructor of Sports Medicine, Department of Physical Medicine and Rehabilitation,
Swedish Spine, Sports and Musculoskeletal Center, Swedish Medical Group, Seattle,
Washington

SCOTT J. PRIMACK, DO
Colorado Rehabilitation and Occupational Medicine, Aurora, Colorado

ETHAN RAND, MD
Sports Medicine Fellow, Department of Rehabilitation and Regenerative Medicine,
Columbia University Medical Center, New York-Presbyterian Hospital, New York,
New York

JACOB L. SELLON, MD
Assistant Professor, Department of Physical Medicine and Rehabilitation, Mayo Clinic
Sports Medicine Center, Mayo Clinic, Rochester, Minnesota

JAY SMITH, MD
Professor, Departments of Physical Medicine and Rehabilitation, Radiology and
Anatomy, Mayo Clinic Sports Medicine Center, Mayo Clinic, Rochester, Minnesota

JEFFREY A. STRAKOWSKI, MD
Clinical Associate Professor, Department of Physical Medicine and Rehabilitation, The
Ohio State University; Associate Director of Medical Education, Department of Physical
Medicine and Rehabilitation, Riverside Methodist Hospital; Director of Musculoskeletal
Research, The McConnell Spine, Sport, and Joint Center, Columbus, Ohio

WALTER I. SUSSMAN, DO
Sports Medicine Fellow, Department of Physical Medicine and Rehabilitation, Emory
University, Atlanta, Georgia

CHRISTOPHER J. VISCO, MD
Associate Professor, Department of Rehabilitation and Regenerative Medicine, Columbia University Medical Center, New York-Presbyterian Hospital, New York, New York

RACHEL WELBEL, MD
Physical Medicine and Rehabilitation Resident, Department of Rehabilitation and Regenerative Medicine, Columbia University Medical Center, New York-Presbyterian Hospital, New York, New York

CHRISTOPHER J. WILLIAMS, MD
Resident, Department of Physical Medicine and Rehabilitation, Emory University, Atlanta, Georgia

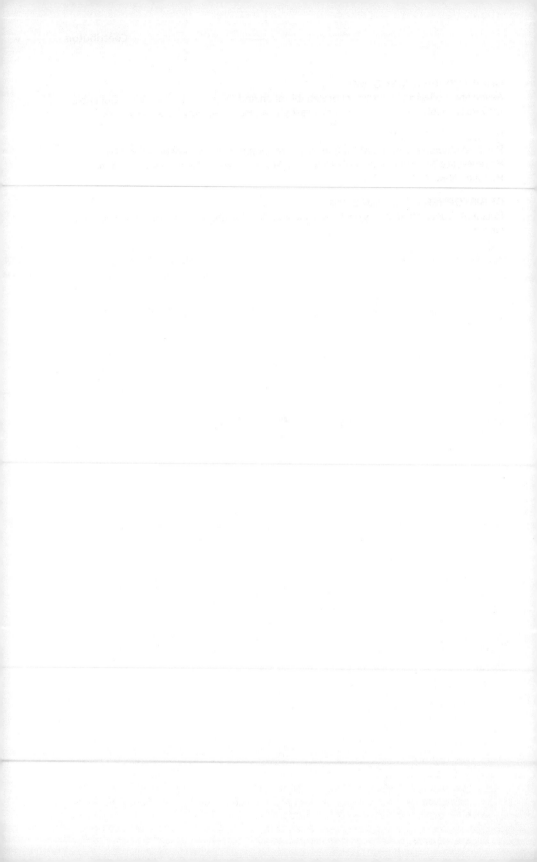

Contents

Ultrasound can be used to guide joint and soft tissue interventions to improve accuracy, efficacy, patient satisfaction, and to minimize complications. This article summarizes the rationale supporting ultrasound-guided injections and explains how to safely and effectively set up and perform these procedures.

 Video content accompanies this article at http://www.pmr.theclinics. com.

Chronic and acute shoulder pain and dysfunction are common complaints among patients. Shoulder pain may be the result of abnormality involving the rotator cuff, subacromial-subdeltoid bursa, biceps tendon, glenoid labrum, glenohumeral joint, acromioclavicular joint, sternoclavicular joint, or glenohumeral joint capsule. Ultrasound-guided (USG) procedures of the shoulder are well established for interventional management. Ultrasound provides the advantages of excellent soft tissue resolution, injection accuracy, low cost, accessibility, portability, lack of ionizing radiation, and the ability to perform real-time image-guided procedures. The purpose of this article is to review common indications and effective techniques for USG injections about the shoulder.

High-resolution ultrasonography can help clinicians visualize key anatomic structures of the elbow and guide periarticular and intra-articular injections. Historically, most procedures done around the elbow have been done using landmark guidance, and few studies have reported the accuracy of ultrasound-guided injections in the elbow region. This article reviews common musculoskeletal disorders about the elbow that can be evaluated with ultrasound, reviews the literature on ultrasound-guided injections of the elbow region, and describes the senior author's preferred approach for the most commonly performed elbow region injections.

injection about the foot and ankle. As much as possible, the procedures described are based on commonly used or published techniques. An in-depth knowledge of the regional anatomy and understanding of different approaches when performing ultrasound-guided procedures allows clinicians to adapt to any clinical scenario.

Mark-Friedrich B. Hurdle

As the population ages, more patients are developing degenerative changes of the spine and associated pain. Although interventional procedures for axial and radicular spine pain have been available for decades, common imaging modalities have relied on ionizing radiation for guidance. Over the past decade, ultrasound has become increasingly popular to image both peripheral musculoskeletal and axial structures. This article reviews the use of ultrasound in the guidance of spine procedures, including cervical and lumbar facet injections and medial branch blocks, third occipital nerve blocks, thoracic facet and costotransverse joint injections, sacroiliac joint injections, and caudal and interlaminar epidural injections.

Jeffrey A. Strakowski

Ultrasound guidance allows real-time visualization of the needle in peripheral nerve procedures, improving accuracy and safety. Sonographic visualization of the peripheral nerve and surrounding anatomy can provide valuable information for diagnostic purposes and procedure enhancement. Common procedures discussed are the suprascapular nerve at the suprascapular notch, deep branch of the radial nerve at the supinator, median nerve at the pronator teres and carpal tunnel, lateral cutaneous nerve of the thigh, superficial fibular nerve at the leg, tibial nerve at the ankle, and interdigital neuroma. For each procedure, the indications, relevant anatomy, preprocedural scanning technique, and injection procedure itself are detailed.

Gerard Malanga, Dena Abdelshahed, and Prathap Jayaram

The application of regenerative therapies for the treatment of musculoskeletal conditions has emerged over the last decade with recent acceleration. These include prolotherapy, platelet-rich plasma, and mesenchymal stem cell therapy. These strategies augment the body's innate physiology to heal pathologic processes. This article presents an overview of platelet-rich plasma and mesenchymal stem cell therapy for the treatment of musculoskeletal injuries. A brief literature review is included, as are techniques for the use of ultrasound guidance to assist with these procedures.

Evan Peck, Elena Jelsing, and Kentaro Onishi

Tendinopathy is increasingly recognized as an important cause of musculoskeletal pain and disability. Tendinopathy is thought to be principally a degenerative process, rather than inflammatory as was traditionally believed. Consequently, traditional tendinopathy treatments focused solely on decreasing inflammation have often been ineffective or even harmful. The advancement of ultrasound for guidance of outpatient musculoskeletal procedures has facilitated the development of novel percutaneous procedures for the treatment of tendinopathy, mostly by using mechanical intervention to stimulate regeneration. Several of these techniques, including percutaneous needle tenotomy, percutaneous ultrasonic tenotomy, high-volume injection, and percutaneous needle scraping, are reviewed in this article.

Scott J. Primack

Musculoskeletal ultrasound has a rich history originally rooted in nautical technology. In recent years, it has proliferated significantly for both diagnostic and interventional purposes in the point-of-care clinical setting by nonradiologist musculoskeletal clinicians. This article outlines the history of musculoskeletal ultrasound, examines present developments, and discusses its future outlook.

PHYSICAL MEDICINE AND REHABILITATION CLINICS OF NORTH AMERICA

VISIT THE CLINICS ONLINE!
Access your subscription at:
www.theclinics.com

Foreword

A New Interventional Field?

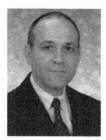

Santos F. Martinez, MD, MS
Consulting Editor

I applaud and thank Dr Peck for this excellent issue on ultrasound-guided procedures, which is a landmark effort bringing together gifted clinicians and researchers to share recent advances. The impact of ultrasound refinement for neuromuscular and sports medicine diagnostic imaging and procedural techniques cannot be overstated. This field has evolved through a combination of technological advances, clinician ingenuity, and market demand for less expensive point-of-care alternatives. The United States was slow to embrace MSK ultrasound in earlier years. Radiologists such as Dr Sofka and Dr Adler from the Hospital for Special Surgery and Dr Nazarian at Thomas Jefferson Hospital had great foresight and were a few of many that were gracious to open their doors to many of us for an introduction to this modality. Dr Jay Smith and Dr Jonathan Finnoff from Mayo Clinic were further instrumental in expanding this exposure among Physiatrists. The landscape of musculoskeletal and sports medicine use of ultrasound has been evolving rapidly, developing into what may be in the future an adjunct subspecialty with many interested fields (physical medicine and rehabilitation, sports medicine, radiology, rheumatology, and so forth). This reminds one of the impact interventional spine specialists made to spine care and interventional cardiology to cardiology. Not only does musculoskeletal interventional ultrasound provide alternative imaging and procedural avenues, but also the evolvement of biocellular medicine is sure to further challenge traditional treatment paradigms. This latter field has drawn considerable attention, is controversial to many, and will be further addressed in depth in the next issue of *Physical Medicine and Rehabilitation Clinics of North America*, the topic of which will be

Phys Med Rehabil Clin N Am 27 (2016) xiii–xiv
http://dx.doi.org/10.1016/j.pmr.2016.06.010
1047-9651/16/$ – see front matter © 2016 Published by Elsevier Inc.

Regenerative Medicine. I hope and suspect that our colleagues will enjoy these two informative treatises.

Santos F. Martinez, MD, MS
Campbell Clinic
Department of Orthopaedics
University of Tennessee
Memphis, TN 38104, USA

E-mail address:
smartinez@campbellclinic.com

Preface

Outpatient Ultrasound-Guided Musculoskeletal Techniques

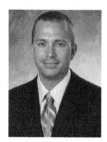

Evan Peck, MD
Editor

I am proud to present this special issue of *Physical Medicine and Rehabilitation Clinics of North America* dedicated to outpatient ultrasound-guided musculoskeletal techniques. Specifically, this issue includes relevant and timely review articles authored by esteemed experts addressing various key topics pertinent to the use of ultrasound guidance for procedures among musculoskeletal clinicians. Common themes throughout the issue are not only the improvement in accuracy, efficacy, and safety of many procedures previously performed without image guidance or with other means of image guidance but also a host of novel interventional techniques not otherwise feasible prior to the use of musculoskeletal ultrasound. In addition to reviewing the pertinent literature related to ultrasound-guided musculoskeletal procedures, this issue also serves as a valuable instruction manual containing thorough but practical information related to procedural performance as well as tips and potential pitfalls.

The first article in the issue addresses fundamental considerations for ultrasound-guided musculoskeletal procedures, including basic ultrasound physics and machine settings; patient, clinician, machine, transducer, and needle positioning; and important safety and technical tips. Six subsequent articles discuss the six major peripheral joint regions commonly encountered in the practice of musculoskeletal ultrasound: shoulder, elbow, wrist and hand, hip, knee, and foot and ankle. For each of these major peripheral body regions, ultrasound-guided aspirations and injections of targets such as joints, bursae, tendon sheaths, and cysts are discussed, including relevant literature and detailed procedural instructions.

Following the discussions of the peripheral joint regions, the focus shifts to the evolving field of ultrasound-guided spine procedures. Although traditionally, most interventional spine procedures have been performed under fluoroscopy, ultrasound possesses unique characteristics that have increased its utilization for spinal procedures, and an article dedicated to that topic is therefore included. Next is an extensive review of ultrasound-guided peripheral nerve procedures.

Phys Med Rehabil Clin N Am 27 (2016) xv–xvi
http://dx.doi.org/10.1016/j.pmr.2016.05.001
1047-9651/16/$ – see front matter © 2016 Published by Elsevier Inc.

Ultrasound-guided procedures for the diagnosis and treatment of peripheral focal nerve entrapments are discussed in that article, including the suprascapular nerve at the suprascapular notch, deep branch of the radial nerve at the supinator, median nerve at both the pronator teres and the carpal tunnel, lateral cutaneous nerve of the thigh, superficial fibular nerve at the leg, tibial nerve at the ankle, and interdigital neuroma.

The use of orthobiologics in musculoskeletal medical practice has expanded commensurate with the increased use of musculoskeletal ultrasound over the past several years. This exciting and rapidly growing area was deserving of its own article in this issue. The delivery of agents such as platelet-rich plasma and mesenchymal stem cells using ultrasound guidance for the treatment of musculoskeletal disorders is covered extensively in that article. The next article in the issue is dedicated to the evolving and increasingly relevant topic of advanced procedures for tendinopathy, most of which have been developed or increased in safety due to the emergence of ultrasound guidance. As our understanding of the pathophysiology of chronic tendon disease has improved, novel procedures have been developed, including percutaneous needle tenotomy, percutaneous ultrasonic tenotomy, high-volume injection, and percutaneous needle scraping. The evidence for and performance of these procedures are explored in detail in that article. The final article in this issue discusses the interesting origins of the use of ultrasound in medicine, a brief history of musculoskeletal ultrasound, its present state and developments, and its future outlook.

I hope that this issue serves as a concise yet complete review of the most practical and current interventional musculoskeletal ultrasound literature for the practicing clinician. In addition, I believe the reader will find valuable procedural tips and instruction, even for the seasoned musculoskeletal ultrasound interventionalist.

Evan Peck, MD
Section of Sports Health
Department of Orthopaedic Surgery
Cleveland Clinic Florida
525 Okeechobee Boulevard, Suite 1400
West Palm Beach, FL 33401, USA

E-mail address:
pecke@ccf.org

Fundamental Considerations for Ultrasound-Guided Musculoskeletal Interventions

Ethan Rand, MD[a], Rachel Welbel, MD[a], Christopher J. Visco, MD[b],*

KEYWORDS

- Image guidance • Injection • Musculoskeletal • Sonography • Ultrasound
- Ultrasound-guided injection

KEY POINTS

- Ultrasound can be used to guide joint and soft tissue interventions to improve accuracy, efficacy, patient satisfaction, and to minimize complications.
- An understanding of ultrasound principles and techniques is critical to performing any ultrasound-guided procedure.
- Appropriate preparation allows the physician to safely and effectively perform ultrasound-guided procedures.

INTRODUCTION

Ultrasound use has expanded exponentially in the musculoskeletal arena in recent years for several reasons, including improved safety, portability, decreased cost, and lack of ionizing radiation.[1] In regard to joint and soft tissue injuries, ultrasound is useful for differentiating between acute injuries, chronic disease, and normal anatomic variations. Further, the practitioner can guide a procedure for the treatment of musculoskeletal disease by following the placement of the needle in real time.[2] However, to appreciate and understand the benefit and rationale of ultrasound-guided (USG) injections, the practitioner must have a basic understanding of the ultrasound machine system.

The process of obtaining an ultrasound image begins with the reverse piezoelectric effect.[3,4] The ultrasound machine sends a pulsed electrical signal to the transducer

[a] Department of Rehabilitation and Regenerative Medicine, Columbia University Medical Center, New York-Presbyterian Hospital, 180 Fort Washington Avenue, Harkness Building 1-167, New York, NY, USA; [b] Department of Rehabilitation and Regenerative Medicine, Columbia University Medical Center, New York-Presbyterian Hospital, 180 Fort Washington Avenue, Harkness Building 1-167, New York, NY 10032, USA
* Corresponding author.
E-mail address: cv2245@cumc.columbia.edu

Phys Med Rehabil Clin N Am 27 (2016) 539–553
http://dx.doi.org/10.1016/j.pmr.2016.04.012
1047-9651/16/$ – see front matter © 2016 Elsevier Inc. All rights reserved.

pmr.theclinics.com

crystals, which transforms that energy into an intermittent acoustic wave, a form of mechanical energy. These sound waves are then transmitted to the tissues via a sonoconductive gel. The acoustic waves interact with tissue and some waves will be reflected back to the transducer, whereas others are absorbed and refracted. The reflected intermittent acoustic waves return to the transducer and are then converted via the direct piezoelectric effect to an electrical signal.[3,4] This electrical signal is then translated into an image on the ultrasound screen. Different transducers with varying crystal properties and thickness determine the frequency of the acoustic wave (see later discussion).[5,6]

Structures that are perpendicular to the transducer will create an angle of insonation of approximately 90°, optimizing the image. Maximizing the reflection produces a bright (hyperechoic) image. Structures with less reflective interfaces will produce a darker (hypoechoic) image. The interface between structures that have very different impedances may also appear hyperechoic, whereas structures with similar impedances may be isoechoic, or of similar echogenicity (overall brightness in sonographic appearance). Furthermore, it is important to realize that ultrasound images are based on the relative material properties of a tissue and its adjacent tissues rather than solely on the properties of that tissue in isolation.[6] Finally, some structures, such as bone, allow no echoes to extend deep to their surfaces and, therefore, the area beneath the surface, or acoustic interface, will appear black from shadowing, also referred to as anechoic (absence of echoes).[5]

Rationale for Ultrasound Guidance for Procedures

Joint and soft tissue injections have been a cornerstone of musculoskeletal medicine and the growth of ultrasound has made many of those injections more accurate and efficacious. Injection accuracy is defined as placing the needle tip and, if desired, injectate into the intended structure.[7] Palpation-guided (PG) injections are more likely to result in adverse effects, including hemarthrosis, septic joint, postinjection pain, and systemic effects.[8] Accuracy may be particularly important when injecting an orthobiologic substance, such as platelet-rich plasma or mesenchymal stem cells, in which precise accuracy of injectate placement is paramount to achievement of its proposed benefit.[1]

Limitations of Palpation-Guided Injections

In addition to potential inaccuracy relative to USG injections, a limitation of PG injections is a possible greater risk of injury to nearby structures. For example, PG injections into the glenohumeral joint are at risk of penetrating the long head of the biceps tendon.[9] Although many clinicians may be confidant in their PG injection technique, many structures are surprisingly difficult to palpate accurately. For example, the accuracy rate for palpation of the biceps tendon in a small group of physicians was only 5%.[10] This investigation found that physicians typically palpated medial to the biceps tendon, often over the subscapularis tendon, making a PG injection in this region potentially unfavorable for both intended therapeutic effect and safety. Furthermore, accuracy rates for PG biceps tendon sheath injections have been found to be 27% compared with 87% with USG injections.[11]

The hip joint is a common source of disease and lies in close proximity to significant neurovascular structures. Injecting the hip joint without imaging carries risk of injury to the femoral nerve, among other vital structures. In PG intra-articular hip injections via the anterior approach, the needle pierced or contacted the femoral nerve in more than a quarter of injections and came within 5 mm in almost two-thirds of the injections.[12]

In the literature, even many superficial, seemingly easy to palpate, structures have poor accuracy rates when injected with a PG technique, and the accuracy of palpation does not always increase with provider experience. In 1 study, physical medicine and rehabilitation resident physicians palpated the acromioclavicular joint with 17% accuracy.[13] The knee is a fairly superficial joint that is often injected without ultrasound guidance. However, ultrasound guidance enables the practitioner to have better visualization of the joint recess, especially in patients with a large body habitus or in the context of degenerative changes that may alter anatomic landmarks. Even in a nonarthritic knee, the accuracy rate for palpation of the lateral knee joint was found to be 58%.[13] The subacromial-subdeltoid bursa is also frequently injected via PG but it has been found that the injectate frequently reaches not only the bursa but also neighboring, potentially unintended structures.[9] For a particularly challenging injection, such as into an interdigital neuroma of the foot, ultrasound guidance ensures accuracy.[7]

Contraindications

There are no contraindications to the use of diagnostic ultrasound. However, general procedural considerations apply, including the use of aseptic technique and use of the as low as reasonably achievable (ALARA) principle, wherein no ultrasound scanning is performed on a patient beyond what is necessary.

Efficacy

Efficacy of USG injections is complex and depends on the outcome scale used, the disease process being treated, the structure injected, individual patient factors, concomitant diagnoses and treatments, and the injectate used. In a group of subjects with inflammatory arthritis, USG injections were more accurate and there was a greater improvement in function if accuracy was improved. However, there was no difference in outcome when comparing USG and PG injections at 2 and 6 weeks following the procedures.[14] This is representative of the idea that extra-articular steroid injections may still be efficacious, due to a regional effect, in patients with inflammatory arthritis.

Studies show USG injections have reduced procedural pain, reduction in pain scores, increase in responder rate, reduction in nonresponder rate, and an increase in therapeutic duration.[15–17] It has been speculated that less procedural pain is secondary to the ability to direct the needle away from pain-sensitive structures while under ultrasound guidance. Further, decreased postprocedural pain is associated with less intra-articular bleeding.[8]

Ultrasound was also associated with increased detection of effusion and increased volume of aspirated fluid.[17] This may result in a decreased number of procedures that are required, exposing the patient to less risk as well as improving the efficacy of the procedure. In a systematic review comparing USG to PG injections, the ultrasound group showed greater short-term improvement.[18]

Although there are limited data on functional outcomes, patient satisfaction plays a large role in efficacy. Glenohumeral joint USG injections were less painful and enable accuracy of 94% compared with 72% with fluoroscopy-guided injections.[19] Injections performed under ultrasound guidance were also associated with better self-reported health-related quality of life.[14]

Cost-Effectiveness

USG injections have shown to result in a cost reduction for patient per year and an even greater reduction is cost for responder per year. In fact, USG injections reduced the cost per patient per year by 8% compared with PG injections.[15] Notably, the cost-effectiveness of USG injections will depend on the skill of the clinician performing the injection, underscoring the need for proper training for those performing these procedures. A clinician with insufficient training in the performance of USG injections may be more likely to perform an inaccurate injection or damage nearby neurovascular structures. Procedural complications may result in pain, discomfort, and more health care expenditure.[7]

Limitations of Ultrasound-Guided Injections

Perhaps the greatest limitation to USG injections is the training, including correct instruction, sufficient practice, and time commitment involved to become a proficient musculoskeletal sonographer. However, as ultrasound training is incorporated into more residency and fellowship curricula, physicians who complete their training will be more proficient in ultrasound. Not only will physicians improve the accuracy and efficacy of standard joint and soft tissue injections, practitioners will be able to expand their injection repertoire. They will be able to perform procedures that were previously considered unsafe or were only done via fluoroscopy, which may be more costly and has more contraindications than ultrasound. For example, specialized tendon procedures, such as percutaneous needle tenotomy, are only feasible and safe because of the development of these techniques using ultrasound guidance. Although some clinicians believe fluoroscopically-guided injections are easier to learn than USG injections, and in many cases provide similar accuracy, fluoroscopy has several drawbacks, including increased costs, radiation exposure, lack of portability, and general lack of availability at the point-of-care or office setting. However, some injections are more safely and effectively performed with fluoroscopic guidance than USG, such as certain spine procedures (see Hurdle MFB: Ultrasound-Guided Spinal Procedures for Pain: A Review, in this issue).

PROCEDURAL CONSIDERATIONS
Preparation

Most USG injections can be performed safely and comfortably in the office setting with common equipment, aseptic technique, and medications (**Fig. 1**). Informed and written consent should be obtained before all procedures, discussing the goals of the procedure, potential benefits, risks, and alternatives.

Patient Positioning

The patient should assume a comfortable position that will facilitate his or her comfort as well as the performance of the injection. When possible, a supine, prone, or lateral decubitus position is preferable to a seated position to avoid injury in the setting of vasovagal syncope. Additionally, the clinician should provide the patient with expectations during each step of preparation and procedure to alleviate any potential anxiety and improve comfort. Some providers offer a video monitor for the patient to watch the ultrasound display without seeing needles, blood, or skin puncture.

Ergonomic Considerations

The height and placement of the examination table, clinician's chair if applicable, and ultrasound machine should be adjusted to maintain an appropriate ergonomically friendly arrangement. Considerations include maintaining proper clinician posture, providing adequate support for the clinician's upper limbs during the procedure to avoid fatigue and improve dexterity, and placement of the ultrasound screen

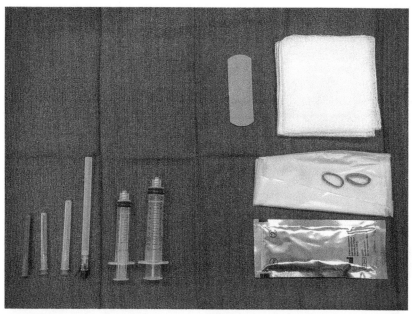

Fig. 1. A sterile tray with common USG procedural materials, including sterile transducer cover, sterile gel, syringe for local anesthesia, syringe for therapeutic medication, blunt fill needle, needle to deliver the local anesthetic, needle to deliver the therapeutic medication, gauze, and a bandage.

approximately 60 cm in front of the clinician. Lighting should be dimmed for comfortable screen viewing. Improper ergonomic setup can lead to overuse injuries for the clinician and can detrimentally affect performance during a procedure. A highly adjustable environment, including the ultrasound machine, clinician's chair, and examination table, improves ergonomics.

Transducer Handling

Appropriately grasping the transducer will help to reduce fatigue, overuse injuries, and is critical for transducer stability during a procedure (**Fig. 2**). A palmar rather than a pincer grip is preferred when holding the transducer. Optimal control and stability of the transducer is obtained by allowing the body of the transducer to rest in the palm because control is achieved using a grip primarily between the thumb, index, and middle fingers. The heel of the palm, along with the ring and little finger, should be in contact with the patient, minimizing the amount of pressure required to place on the transducer. When scanning, avoid using gloves, which decrease the coefficient of friction and increase the hand pressure. With less pressure needed to stabilize the transducer, the clinician is able to improve image optimization, patient comfort, and reduce tissue displacement.

Preprocedural Scanning

Once the appropriate preprocedural setup is obtained, a preprocedural ultrasound scan should always be performed to identify the normal, abnormal, unexpected, or undesired structures or conditions that may be found. The preprocedural scan initially is used to confirm diagnostic findings, visualize and optimize the image of the structural

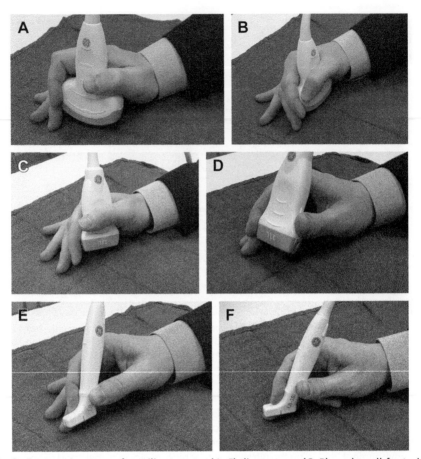

Fig. 2. Ergonomic grasps of curvilinear-array (*A, B*), linear-array (*C, D*), and small-footprint linear-array (hockey-stick) (*E, F*) ultrasound transducers.

targets, and identify sonographic landmarks. It is also used to identify anatomic variations, structures to avoid, and assess for potential contraindications or reasons to abort or delay the procedure. If concerning findings are seen on the prescan (eg, mass), the procedure can be deferred and additional workup can be performed as indicated. The clinician may also trial various transducers and ultrasound machine settings before the procedure, as these adjustments may be more cumbersome once sterile preparation is performed and injection materials are prepared. Identification of adjacent neurovascular structures is critical. Use of color and power Doppler imaging can be helpful.

Transducer Selection

The first step in optimizing an ultrasound image is selecting the appropriate transducer. Generally, most USG procedures can be performed using a high-frequency (>10 MHz) linear-array transducer; however, for more superficial or deeper targets a small-footprint very-high-frequency (>15 MHz) linear array (hockey-stick) or low-frequency (<10 MHz) curvilinear transducer may be used, respectively. The small profile and high frequencies used by the hockey-stick transducer can provide greater spatial resolution of superficial structures and the ability to easily bring the injection site closer to the target, particularly on uneven areas with bony prominences, such as in the hand or foot. The curvilinear transducer, on the other hand, has a larger profile, uses lower frequencies, and is ideally used for accessing deeper structures, such as those around the hip region.

Instrumentation and Other Variables

Frequency

Each transducer is capable of operating within a certain frequency range, typically expressed as megahertz, as previously noted. The specific frequency can be further adjusted on the ultrasound machine, balancing spatial resolution and depth of penetration.

Depth

Depth should be adjusted to minimize wasted space on the display while maintaining all structures of interest within the field. Generally, a maximal depth on the ultrasound screen of 1 cm or less beyond the target structure is a reasonable starting point.

Focal zones

Focal zones represent the narrowest portions of the ultrasound beam, and they may be adjusted in number and position along the depth of the display. Focal zones should be placed at the level of interest on the screen. The number of focal zones should be minimized before an intervention to reduce the processing demands and thereby maintain the temporal resolution needed to perform the procedure optimally, that is, the number of focal zones is inversely proportional to frame rate.

Doppler

Color and power Doppler imaging displays movement by detecting the difference between the frequency of the signal transmitted and the signal received by the transducer. Color Doppler adds direction (typically a red or blue scale) revealing motion (toward or away) relative to the transducer. Power Doppler is generally more sensitive for flow but does not provide directional information relative to the transducer. A Doppler examination should be strongly considered during the preprocedural scan to identify and avoid any vascular structures during the subsequent procedure. This is particularly true when a known vascular structure exists near the planned needle approach.

Gain

Gain can be adjusted to brighten the image. When adjusting the gain, regions beyond bone, fluid within vessels, and simple fluid collections should remain nearly anechoic, that is, appear black. Because attenuation of the ultrasound signal often results in the deeper portion of the display, appearing darker than the superficial section, the practitioner can preferentially adjust the gain at varying depths, known as the time gain compensation or depth gain compensation.

Although some ultrasound machines will permit the user to adjust each of these variables independently, others will automatically adjust many of these settings. Additionally, most machines have imaging presets programmed for each region of the body (eg, shoulder or knee presets), with all of these variables adjusted to optimize visualization of those regions. Even when using presets, however, adjustments will need to be made and an understanding of instrumentation and image optimization is crucial for procedural performance.

Artifacts

Angle of incidence or insonation and anisotropy

The angle of incidence (AOI) refers to the angle of the ultrasound beam relative to the structure being visualized. When the angle of the wave relative to the tissue is not perpendicular, that is, AOI is not 90°, a portion of the wave may be directed away from the transducer, thereby creating artifactual attenuation. This artifact, known as anisotropy, commonly appears with dense and uniform tissues, such as tendons, and may be resolved by manipulating the transducer into a more perpendicular orientation relative to the structure. More heterogeneous and less dense tissues, such as nerves, are less prone to anisotropy, and adipose essentially lacks anisotropy. The practitioner can use this principle to optimize the image with regard to anisotropy to aid in tissue differentiation, to improve needle visualization, and diagnostically to further investigate hypoechoic regions of concern for fluid collections or possible muscle, tendon, or ligamentous tear.

Shadowing

Shadowing occurs when reflection of the beam is increased and further penetration is thereby limited. Increased reflection of ultrasound occurs at tissue interfaces, particularly between tissues of varying densities. Particularly at these interfaces, for instance with soft tissue overlying bone, there is increased deep shadowing.

Refractile shadowing

Refractile shadowing is similar in appearance to shadowing artifact; however, it occurs when the ultrasound beam approaches a target at an oblique angle, for instance over the curved surfaces of a transverse tendon.

Reverberation

Reverberation is caused by the repeated detection of a signal from a highly reflective substance such as metal, prosthesis, or bone. This may cause a ring-down effect, appearing as though the structure or substance is occurring repeatedly deeper in the image. Needles are particularly prone to this effect when placed parallel to the transducer.

Posterior acoustic enhancement

Posterior acoustic enhancement or enhanced through-transmission is the result of signal processing to account for signal attenuation with increased tissue depths. Because all tissues do not attenuate the signal equally, tissues deep to tissues that are less absorptive will appear hyperechoic, for example, deep to fluid. A tendon will appear more hyperechoic than if no fluid collection were superficial to it.

Transducer Movements

Translation or sliding involves movement of the transducer relative to the target structure along the skin. Rotation of the transducer is primarily used to alternate between transverse and longitudinal views of a given structure by rotating 90° during a procedure to optimize visualization of the entire needle. Heel-toe movement involves angling the transducer along its long-axis and often requires placing more or less pressure through 1 side of the transducer. This maneuver is important for improving needle visualization by adjusting the AOI. Toggle (ie, tilt or wag) is accomplished by angling the transducer along its short axis and is also an important maneuver when adjusting the AOI. Angling the transducer is also an important part of the preprocedural scan to fully assess all facets of the target structure. Compression involves increasing or decreasing pressure through the transducer into the tissues examined. Compression can be used to displace fluid, compress blood vessels, and can dynamically aid in differentiating between fascial planes.

Identify Optimal Approach

The goal in selecting the optimal approach is to create the safest, shortest path to the target structure. Safety is ensured by avoiding blood vessels, nerves, tendons, and other structures that can potentially be damaged by the needle or injectate. Additionally, the practitioner must consider how to orient the transducer relative to the target and the needle relative to the transducer.

Orientation of transducer to target

Given the versatility and limited field of view of ultrasound, the orientation of transducer to target is generally described in relation to the targeted structure, rather than an anatomic plane, as in computed tomography scan and MRI. Longitudinal (long-axis) views are obtained with the transducer parallel to the structure, whereas transverse (short-axis) views are obtained with the transducer perpendicular to the structure. **Fig. 3** demonstrates longitudinal and transverse orientation of the transducer over the median nerve.

Orientation of needle to transducer

An in-plane approach maintains the long axis of the transducer parallel to the long axis of the needle. Generally, an in-plane approach for injections is the preferred technique because the entire needle shaft, tip, and target are visualized throughout the procedure. The major limitation of in-plane procedures is limited access to superficial targets. The stand-off technique may be used to address this limitation and gain access to superficial structures while maintaining an in-plane approach (**Fig. 4**). A heel-toe maneuver is performed, lifting 1 end of the transducer off the skin, and sterile gel is placed under this portion of the transducer (assuming sterile transducer cover is present and patient is already prepared in a sterile fashion). The needle is then advanced and visualized within the gel before piercing the skin.

The out-of-plane approach places the long axis of the needle perpendicular to the long axis of the transducer, and may be used on several anatomic sites that are not as conducive to in-plane injections, for example, the acromioclavicular joint. This approach may use a walk-down technique wherein the tip of the needle is initially placed superficially under the center of the transducer (**Fig. 5**). Once the tip is visualized, the needle is slightly withdrawn and subsequently advanced with a steeper trajectory. This maneuver is repeated until the target is reached. The major risk involved in using an out-of-plane approach involves uncertainty regarding the depth of needle advancement because the needle tip appears similar to the shaft of the needle. It is of

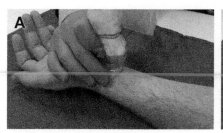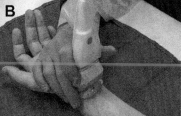

Fig. 3. Demonstration of longitudinal orientation (*A*) and transverse orientation (*B*) of the ultrasound transducer with respect to the median nerve at the wrist.

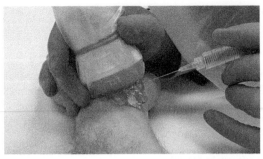

Fig. 4. An in-plane USG injection around the median nerve using the stand-off technique.

paramount importance that the clinician always stops needle advancement once the needle is sonographically visualized while using an out-of-plane injection approach.

During the preprocedural scan, the starting point and site of initial puncture can also be marked, indicating the area surrounding the site that should be prepared in a sterile fashion and as a relatively precise reminder for where to begin the procedure. It may also be helpful to draw a line indicating the initial direction of approach for the injection. Finally, the preprocedural scan provides the clinician with the ability to gauge the depth and length of needle required to perform the procedure, as well as the optimal angle of needle trajectory.

Needle Selection

The needle type, gauge, and length selected depend on the goal of the procedure and preprocedural scan findings. In general, a thinner needle is advisable to reduce procedural discomfort. However, a larger-gauge needle may be necessary for an aspiration or to inject more viscous substances. Longer needles are required for deep structures, such as the hip joint. A needle that is both long and thin may be more prone to deflection as it is advanced, which can be more difficult to control.

Sterility and General Procedural Safety

Every effort should be made to reduce infection. Ideally, aseptic technique should be maintained throughout the procedure. The injection site should be cleaned with

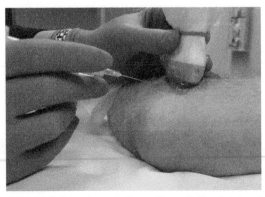

Fig. 5. An out-of-plane USG injection of the radiocapitellar joint using the walk-down technique.

appropriate antimicrobial solution. Transducers should be cleaned between each procedure. Each ultrasound manufacturer should be contacted to identify the recommended cleanser for the machine and transducer.

Materials

The 2014 American Institute for Ultrasound in Medicine (AIUM) Practice Guideline for the Performance of Selected Ultrasound-Guided Procedures notes that "the use of sterile drapes, sterile probe covers, and sterile ultrasound gel may provide the best method to reduce the risk of contamination and infection" (**Fig. 6**).[20] Alternatively, some practitioners use a sterile occlusive dressing to cover the ultrasound transducer face.[20]

Local Anesthesia

Use of local anesthetic can reduce procedural discomfort, particularly when using thick needles (<25 gauge) and can provide an assessment of needle trajectory. Subcutaneous tissue along the needle path can be anesthetized so that the subsequent procedural needle can be advanced with less patient discomfort.

Image Optimization for Needle Guidance

USG procedures should be performed with real-time, continuous visualization of the target structure and needle tip. If the needle tip or the target structure is not visualized, then the needle should not be advanced until relocated and an appropriate trajectory is reestablished. The clinician should only move 1 hand at a time, either that on the needle or on the transducer, but not both simultaneously.

Needle Optimization Techniques

Visualization of the needle depends on gauge and AOI of the ultrasound beam. Optimal detection of the needle will occur when oriented perpendicular to the ultrasound beam (parallel to the transducer). **Fig. 7** demonstrates how a steeper needle trajectory can result in an unfavorable AOI. With a relatively perpendicular needle-ultrasound beam relationship, most of the resultant signal reflects back to the transducer and the needle appears hyperechoic and is readily visualized. The needle is also more obvious with a larger diameter needle. However, this effect is subtle and choice of needle gauge should be determined by procedural need, not improved visualization.

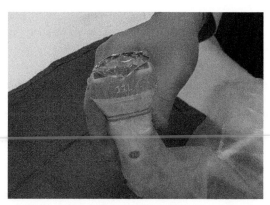

Fig. 6. A linear-array ultrasound transducer with sterile cover and gel.

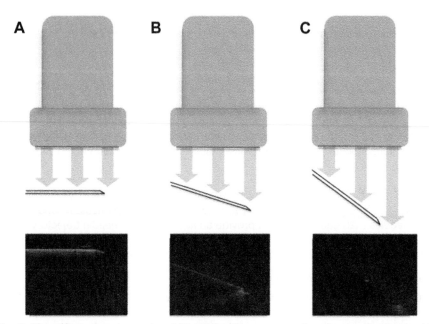

Fig. 7. The effect of an increasing AOI (*A–C*) with corresponding decreased sonographic conspicuity of the needle.

Maintaining favorable orientation of the needle relative to the transducer can be achieved through careful choice of puncture site, adjusting the depth of the needle trajectory, or by performing a heel-toe maneuver. Additional methods include rotation of the needle, slight back-and-forth movements of the needle (ie, jiggle), or injection of a small amount of fluid (eg, anesthetic or saline). Many ultrasound machines also include needle visualization software, designed to improve needle detection; however, when performed with proper technique this software is rarely necessary for needle visualization.

Needle and Target Location Maneuvers

There are several techniques to relocate the needle tip during a free-hand USG procedure. These techniques combine multiple movements discussed previously.

Lock and spin
Translate the transducer until a portion of the needle is identified, then lock in place the part of the transducer over the needle and begin slowly rotating the remaining transducer to completely align the needle with the transducer.

Rhombolocation
The rhombolocation technique is often used for needle fenestration to pass the needle through multiple sections along a plane of tissue (eg, plantar fascia). Following the first successful pass, the needle is partially retracted (without exiting the skin) and, subsequently, the transducer is translated and rotated to the next target. The needle can then be oriented in-plane to the transducer and advanced again through the tissue along the new trajectory.

Lock and rock
This technique creates dynamic resolution of the AOI using a curvilinear transducer by locking it in place over the target, and rocking the transducer, using a heel-toe

maneuver, to maintain the needle tip in a perpendicular relationship with the ultrasound beam.

Tip-toe toggle

Useful during the preprocedural scan, particularly in the setting of tendinopathy to find all calcific and tendinopathic areas. Translate the transducer in short axis along a long tendon in small increments and, with every small incremental advancement (tip-toe), create a toggling motion with the transducer thus decreasing anisotropy of the structure.

Probe-slip, hub-grip, syringe-swap

Allow the transducer to slip into the palm, freeing the first 2 digits to grip the needle hub. Swap the syringe. Return the transducer to the original hand position. This is particularly helpful when a syringe swap is needed while performing an aseptic injection with only 2 hands.

DOCUMENTATION
Procedure Note

Documentation of the procedure should follow the AIUM Practice Guideline for Documentation of an Ultrasound Examination.[21] Procedural documentation should include patient name and identification, facility name, performing provider, date and time of procedure, procedure type, site and laterality, indication for procedure, justification for use of ultrasound, documentation of informed consent, documentation of compliance with the Joint Commission Universal Protocol, documentation of sterile preparation, description of preprocedural scan of the target and associated structures, description of the essential elements of the procedure, including orientation of the transducer to target and needle to transducer, injectate used, needle type and gauge, specimens removed if applicable, complications, and postprocedure care instructions.[21]

Images and Videos

Ideally, ultrasound images or videos of the preprocedural scan, procedure itself, and postprocedure target, associated structures, and at least 1 image of the needle at target site should be saved and labeled appropriately.[21] At minimum, 1 image of the needle placed at the target site is required. Images should be annotated with laterality, site, and orientation of transducer to target (eg, right biceps brachii long head short axis). When appropriate, arrows can be used to mark structures and measurements can be performed (eg, cross-sectional area of the median nerve). Additionally, all images should include the patient identification, facility, and date. Images should be archived and easily retrievable.[21]

SUMMARY

Ultrasound guidance allows the real time visualization of the target, needle, and injectate. A safe and effective USG procedure can be performed by a skilled practitioner aware of the limitations, procedural indications, and understanding of the transducer and equipment. Improved accuracy and efficacy have been reported for many USG procedures versus PG procedures, and a prepared practitioner will be able to adjust the procedure using needle location maneuvers. Aseptic technique requires additional attention to material management and transducer handling, suitable for most office-based applications. The advancement of ultrasound technology and the proliferation of ultrasound training and techniques dictate that it will continue to have an important role in musculoskeletal medicine.

REFERENCES

1. Hoeber S, Aly A-R, Ashworth N, et al. Ultrasound-guided hip joint injections are more accurate than landmark-guided injections: a systematic review and meta-analysis. Br J Sports Med 2015;50:1–5.
2. Daley EL, Bajaj S, Bisson LJ, et al. Improving injection accuracy of the elbow, knee, and shoulder: does injection site and imaging make a difference? A systematic review. Am J Sports Med 2011;39:656–62.
3. Dineva P, Gross D, Muller R, et al. Dynamic fracture of piezoelectric materials: solution of time-harmonic problems via BIEM, 1st ed, solid mechanics and its applications. Cham, Switzerland: Springer International Publishing; 2014.
4. Cerda RM. Understanding quartz crystals and oscillators, Artech house microwave library. Boston (MA): Artech House; 2014.
5. Jacobson JA. Fundamentals of musculoskeletal ultrasound. 2nd edition. Philadelphia: Saunders, Elsevier Inc; 2013.
6. Smith J, Finnoff JT. Diagnostic and interventional musculoskeletal ultrasound: part 1. Fundamentals. PM R 2009;1:64–75.
7. Finnoff JT, Hall MM, Adams E, et al. American Medical Society for Sports Medicine (AMSSM) position statement: interventional musculoskeletal ultrasound in sports medicine. PM R 2015;7:151–68.e12.
8. Berkoff DJ, Miller LE, Block JE. Clinical utility of ultrasound guidance for intra-articular knee injections: a review. Clin Interv Aging 2012;7:89–95.
9. Hall MM. The accuracy and efficacy of palpation versus image-guided peripheral injections in sports medicine. Curr Sports Med Rep 2013;12:296–303.
10. Gazzillo GP, Finnoff JT, Hall MM, et al. Accuracy of palpating the long head of the biceps tendon: an ultrasonographic study. PM R 2011;3:1035–40.
11. Hashiuchi T, Sakurai D, Morimoto M, et al. Accuracy of the biceps tendon sheath injection: ultrasound-guided of unguided injection? A randomized controlled trial. J Shoulder Elbow Surg 2011;20:1069–73.
12. Leopold S, Battista V, Oliverio JA. Safety and efficacy of intraarticular hip injection using anatomic landmarks. Clin Orthop 2001;391:192–7.
13. Rho ME, Chu SK, Yang A, et al. Resident accuracy of joint line palpation using ultrasound verification. PM R 2014;6:920–5.
14. Cunnington J, Marshall N, Hide G, et al. A randomized, double-blind, controlled study of ultrasound-guided corticosteroid injection into the joint of patients with inflammatory arthritis. Arthritis Rheum 2010;62:1862–9.
15. Sibbitt WJ, Band P, Kettwich L, et al. A randomized controlled trial evaluating the cost-effectiveness of sonographic guidance for intra-articular injection of the osteoarthritic knee. J Clin Rheumatol 2011;17:409–15.
16. Sibbitt WJ, Kettwich L, Band P, et al. Does ultrasound guidance improve the outcomes of arthrocentesis and corticosteroid injection of the knee? Scand J Rheumatol 2012;41:66–72.
17. Sibbitt WJ, Peisajovich A, Michael A, et al. Does sonographic needle guidance affect the clinical outcome of intraarticular injections? J Rheumatol 2009;36:1892–902.
18. D'Agostino M-A, Schmidt WA. Ultrasound-guided injections in rheumatology: Actual knowledge on efficacy and procedures. Best Pract Res Clin Rheumatol 2013;27:283–94.

19. Rutten M, Collins J, Maresch B, et al. Glenohumeral joint injection: a comparative study of ultrasound and fluoroscopically guided techniques before MR arthrography. Eur Radiol 2009;19:722–30.
20. American Institute of Ultrasound in Medicine. AIUM practice parameter for the performance of selected ultrasound-guided procedures. Laurel (MD): American Institute of Ultrasound in Medicine; 2014. Available at: http://www.aium.org/resources/statements.aspx.
21. American Institute of Ultrasound in Medicine. AIUM practice parameter for documentation of an ultrasound examination. Laurel (MD): American Institute of Ultrasound in Medicine; 2014. Available at: http://www.aium.org/resources/statements.aspx.

Ultrasound-Guided Interventional Procedures About the Shoulder
Anatomy, Indications, and Techniques

Adam M. Pourcho, DO[a], Sean W. Colio, MD[a],
Mederic M. Hall, MD[b],*

KEYWORDS

- Ultrasound • Ultrasound guidance • Shoulder • Tendinopathy • Bursitis
- Adhesive capsulitis

KEY POINTS

- Diagnosis and treatment of shoulder conditions can prove challenging, and ultrasound allows for precise diagnosis and potential treatment at point of care.
- Ultrasound guidance increases accuracy of injections about the shoulder.
- A detailed understanding of shoulder anatomy is required for safe and effective ultrasound-guided procedures about the shoulder.

 Video content accompanies this article at http://www.pmr.theclinics.com.

INTRODUCTION

The shoulder complex is susceptible to a wide range of traumatic and atraumatic pathologic conditions. Secondary to the relatively superficial location of the anatomic structures of the shoulder, many clinicians use ultrasound (US) for diagnostic and interventional purposes about the shoulder. The increased use of US in the last decade is partially attributed to its portability, low cost compared with MRI, lack of ionizing radiation, and potential increased accuracy and efficacy of procedures versus using palpation guidance.[1–5]

Disclosures: The authors have nothing to disclose.
[a] Department of Physical Medicine and Rehabilitation, Swedish Spine, Sports and Musculoskeletal Center, Swedish Medical Group, 1600 E. Jefferson Street, Suite 300, Seattle, WA 98122, USA; [b] Department of Orthopaedics and Rehabilitation, Radiology, and Family Medicine, University of Iowa Sports Medicine Center, 2701 Prairie Meadow Drive, Iowa City, IA 52242, USA
* Corresponding author.
E-mail address: mederic-hall@uiowa.edu

Phys Med Rehabil Clin N Am 27 (2016) 555–572
http://dx.doi.org/10.1016/j.pmr.2016.04.001
1047-9651/16/$ – see front matter © 2016 Elsevier Inc. All rights reserved.

Multiple pathologic processes about the shoulder can be evaluated with US, including subacromial-subdeltoid (SASD) bursopathy, acromioclavicular joint (ACJ) and sternoclavicular joint (SCJ) arthropathy and synovitis, adhesive capsulitis, long head of the biceps brachii (LHBBT) tendinopathy and tenosynovitis, and rotator cuff (RTC) abnormality, including calcific tendinopathy. Both diagnostic and interventional US are operator-dependent modalities. As such, clinical experience and knowledge of anatomy are essential components to a proper diagnosis and accurate procedure.[2]

In this article, an overview, including anatomy, indications, and techniques for common ultrasound-guided (USG) procedures about the shoulder, is provided.

General procedural setup key points

- A sterile procedural setup with sterile technique, probe covers, and sterile gel is recommended, but recognize that some clinicians may choose to only sterilize the needle puncture site.
- It is important to consider proper ergonomics before performing the procedure, including putting the US machine in front of the practitioner, proper patient positioning, and adjustments to table and chair heights.
- After obtaining an optimal preprocedural image of the target, marking the transducer edges with a surgical marking pen is recommended to allow for efficient reacquisition of the target image after sterile preparation. This procedure is especially useful for novice practitioners.
- Needle selection may vary per clinician preferences and patient factors. Selection of the smallest-gauge needle with the appropriate length for the desired injection is recommended. The needle gauges mentioned in this article are the authors' preferences; in general, smaller gauges are more comfortable for the patient and are typically well visualized with US about the shoulder with good technique.
- Injection contents and respective amounts will vary between practitioners and depend on the goals of the procedure.

SUBACROMIAL/SUBDELTOID BURSA

The SASD bursa is a potential synovial space that lies deep to the deltoid muscle, acromion, and the coracoacromial ligament, and superficial to the supraspinatus tendon, rotator interval (RI), greater tuberosity, and intertubercular groove.[1] The SASD extends approximately 3 cm lateral over the deltoid shelf of the greater tuberosity of the humerus and is surrounded by peribursal fat, which is sonographically hyperechoic relative to the anechoic bursa.[6] The normal bursa is about 1 mm in thickness and located just deep to the more superficial layer of peribursal fat.[6]

SASD bursopathy, a condition that may be a primary or secondary cause of pain, is the most commonly reported finding on diagnostic US of the painful shoulder.[7] Given its superficial location, the bursa is best visualized using a high-frequency (>10 MHz) linear-array transducer placed long axis to the supraspinatus tendon fibers. Sonographic findings of bursal enlargement with anechoic fluid or soft tissue hypertrophy are common in the setting of bursopathy[8] and may be accompanied by hyperemia on color Doppler. These findings can be confirmed as symptomatic on physical examination with provocative maneuvers, such as the Neer and Hawkins impingement tests, and on dynamic US with painful bunching of the bursa under the acromion as the humerus is abducted.[7,8]

It has been established that impingement of the SASD bursa can lead to bursopathy, which can be painful and debilitating, especially to patients who perform repetitive overhead activities.[8] SASD bursal injections are commonly used for both diagnostic and therapeutic purposes.[9–11] Cadaveric studies on palpation-guided (PG) injections report accuracy rates ranging from 29% to 83%.[12–16] Two studies comparing the accuracy rate of USG injections versus PG injections demonstrated accuracy rates from 65% to 100% when using USG.[17,18] It has been demonstrated that short- and long-term relief of shoulder pain secondary to subacromial impingement can be gained with SASD bursa injections.[9,10]

AUTHORS' PREFERRED TECHNIQUE FOR ULTRASOUND-GUIDED SUBACROMIAL-SUBDELTOID BURSA INJECTION

Positioning for the lateral approach to the SASD bursa involves placing the patient in the lateral decubitus position on the contralateral side (**Fig. 1**A). A high-frequency (>10 MHz) linear-array transducer is placed long axis to the supraspinatus tendon (anatomic coronal plane) to visualize the SASD bursa. Once localized deep to the deltoid and peribursal fat, a 25-gauge 38-mm needle (or in larger patients, a 25-gauge 51-mm needle) is introduced in an in-plane lateral-to-medial fashion under direct USG to anesthetize the skin and needle path into the SASD bursa (**Fig. 1**B). A small amount of lidocaine can be used to confirm flow within the bursa. The syringe is exchanged, and after sonographic confirmation of needle tip placement, the SASD bursa is injected under direct USG with the desired amount of injectate (usually 3–5 mL) (Video 1).

ACROMIOCLAVICULAR JOINT

The ACJ is the articulation between the lateral hyaline-covered clavicle and the medial hyaline-covered acromion. The ACJ has a centrally located fibrocartilaginous disc, which can partially or completely separate the joint into medial and lateral joint cavities.[1,6] The ACJ is stabilized by several important ligaments. Laterally, the ACJ is stabilized by the inferior and superior ACJ ligaments, the latter of which has contributing fibers from the coracoacromial ligament.[19] Medially, the joint is stabilized by the

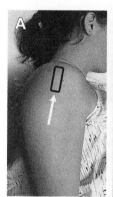
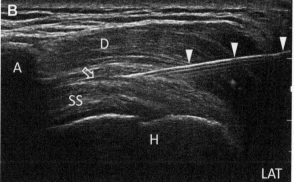

Fig. 1. US-guided SASD bursa injection. (*A*) With the patient in the lateral decubitus position on the contralateral side, with the ipsilateral arm placed on the hip, the transducer (*rectangle*) is placed long axis to the supraspinatus tendon. The needle trajectory (*solid arrow*) is in-plane using a lateral-to-medial approach. (*B*) US image arranged with lateral to the right of the image, demonstrating correct placement of the needle (*arrowheads*) tip within the SASD bursa (*open arrow*). See also Video 1.

coracoclavicular ligaments (conoid and trapezoid), which also limit vertical displacement of the clavicle relative to the acromion.[19]

The ACJ is commonly affected by both idiopathic and posttraumatic disorders, and degenerative changes are also a common cause of pain.[19,20] However, degenerative changes of the ACJ are also frequently seen in asymptomatic individuals over the age of 35 years.[20–22] Given the high prevalence of ACJ degeneration in asymptomatic individuals, identification of the ACJ as the primary pain generator in individuals with shoulder pain can prove challenging. Physical examination maneuvers, pain referral patterns, and imaging findings have been shown to lack sensitivity and specificity when identifying the ACJ as the primary pain generator.[23,24]

As a very superficial structure, the ACJ is best visualized using a high-frequency (>10 MHz) linear-array transducer placed long axis (anatomic coronal plane) to the clavicle and acromion. A hypoechoic intra-articular disc may be visualized within the joint as well as up to 3 mm of physiologic anechoic joint capsule distension.[25] Common US findings of abnormality at the ACJ include widening or instability of the joint (ACJ separation), cortical irregularities, joint effusion with synovitis or capsular distension, and possible ganglion cysts (**Fig. 2**B, C).[6,7]

Some investigators have suggested the use of injections to help diagnose and assist in clinical decision-making in patients with apparent ACJ pain.[15,24,26,27] Despite its superficial location, the accuracy of PG ACJ injections has been reportedly low, with

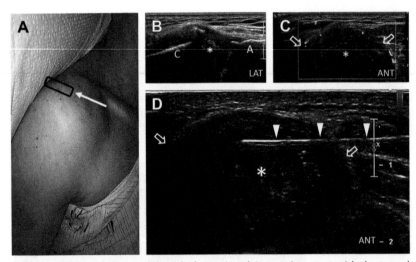

Fig. 2. US-guided ACJ injection. (A) With the patient lying supine, start with the transducer (*rectangle*) over the clavicle in an oblique sagittal plane and translate laterally until the bony acoustic landmark of the clavicle disappears. Slight "wagging" of the transducer tail will produce image seen in (C and D). The needle trajectory (*solid arrow*) is from anterior to posterior via an in-plane technique. (B) By turning the transducer 90° to an oblique coronal plane, a long-axis view of the ACJ (*asterisk*) is visualized with LAT to the right of the image. In this example, the patient has inflammatory arthropathy with hyperechoic osteophytes and capsular distension. (C) By orienting the transducer in the same fashion as (A), a long-axis view of the same patient's ACJ (*asterisk*) is produced with ANT to the right of the image. Notice the hyperemia in the joint capsule (*open arrows*) on low-flow color Doppler, indicating active synovitis. (D) US image with ANT to the right demonstrating the in-plane anterior-to-posterior view of the hyperechoic needle (*arrowheads*) within the joint capsule (*open arrows*) of the ACJ (*asterisk*). See also Video 2.

accuracy rates ranging from 40% to 72%.[15,28–31] Conversely, USG injections have reported accuracy rates of 90% to 100% in both clinical and cadaveric studies.[28–30,32]

AUTHORS' PREFERRED TECHNIQUE FOR ULTRASOUND-GUIDED ACROMIOCLAVICULAR JOINT INJECTION

For the anterior in-plane approach to the ACJ, the patient is placed in the supine position with a few pillows under the upper back or the head of the examination table elevated (**Fig. 2**A). A high-frequency (>10 MHz) linear-array transducer is placed short axis to the clavicle and moved laterally until the bony acoustic landmarks of the clavicle disappear (**Fig. 2**A, C, D). Once the ACJ is localized using the technique above, a 27-gauge 32-mm needle is introduced in an in-plane anterior-to-posterior fashion under direct USG to anesthetize the skin and needle path into the ACJ (see **Fig. 2**D). Following correct placement, the syringe is exchanged, positioning is reconfirmed sonographically, and the ACJ is injected under USG with the desired amount of injectate (usually <1 mL) (Video 2). Care must be taken to avoid excess distension of the joint because this can result in pain after the procedure. Given the relatively small size of the joint, clinicians should be cognizant of the procedural goals, whether diagnostic or therapeutic. This injection can also be performed with an out-of-plane approach similar to that described later in the SCJ injection section of this article.

STERNOCLAVICULAR JOINT INJECTIONS

The SCJ is composed of the hyaline-covered sternal end of the clavicle and the hyaline-covered clavicular notch of the manubrium and first rib, separated by an intra-articular disc.[33–35] It represents the only articulation between the axial skeleton and the upper limb. The SCJ is stabilized medially by the anterior and posterior sternoclavicular ligaments and laterally by the interclavicular and costoclavicular ligaments.[34,36] Additional stability is provided by a complete or incomplete intra-articular disc, which is contiguous with both the sternoclavicular and the interclavicular ligaments.[35]

Although uncommon, the SCJ can be a clinically important source of shoulder pain. The SCJ can be affected by both idiopathic and posttraumatic arthritis, dislocation or subluxation, synovitis-acne-pustulosis-hyperostosis-osteitis, avascular necrosis (Friedrich disease), rheumatic arthritis, and crystalline arthropathies.[37–43] The pain referral pattern for the SCJ is widespread and often nonspecific.[44] Furthermore, degeneration of the SCJ and intra-articular disc is common with advanced aged and often asymptomatic.[35,45] Therefore, it can be clinically challenging to determine if the SCJ is the primary pain generator in a patient presenting with shoulder or even anterior neck pain.

As another superficial structure, the SCJ is best visualized using a high-frequency (>10 MHz) linear-array transducer placed long axis to the clavicle (short axis to the joint). A hypoechoic intra-articular disc may be visualized within the joint, which can be accentuated by increasing the gain. Common pathologic findings on US evaluation include cortical irregularities, capsular distension, and hyperemia on low-flow color Doppler in the case of synovitis (**Fig. 3**B).[7,46,47]

Some clinicians have advocated for the use of diagnostic and therapeutic injections into the SCJ to assist in clinical decision-making and to treat symptomatic patients.[38,42,46,48,49] PG injections of the SCJ have a reported accuracy rate of 74% to 78%.[50] Clinicians have also used fluoroscopic and computed tomographic guidance for injection and aspiration of the SCJ with reported good clinical outcomes.[48,49,51] In

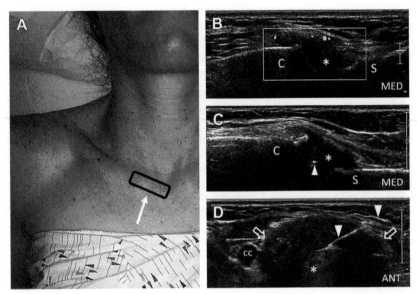

Fig. 3. US-guided SCJ injection. (*A*) With the patient lying supine, the transducer (*rectangle*) is placed over the SCJ in an oblique axial plane with the center of the joint placed in the center of the transducer. The needle trajectory (*solid arrow*) is via an out-of-plane, anterior-to-posterior approach. (*B*) Long-axis US image of a patient's right SCJ (*asterisk*), demonstrating active inflammatory arthropathy. Note the hyperemia on low-flow color Doppler, indicating active synovitis. (*C*) US image demonstrating the hyperechoic needle tip (*arrowhead*) introduced via an out-of-plane trajectory within the center of the SCJ (*asterisk*). (*D*) By turning the transducer 90° to the orientation demonstrated in (*A*), a long axis of the needle (*arrowheads*) can be seen within in the center of the SCJ (*asterisk*). *Open arrows* identify the joint capsule. Note the common carotid (CC) artery lies directly posterior to the SCJ and represents a potential complication to the injection. This injection may also be done via an in-plane approach similar to that described in the ACJ section of this article. See also Video 3.

one cadaveric study, the USG success rate was 100% using an out-of-plane technique.[52]

AUTHORS' PREFERRED TECHNIQUE FOR ULTRASOUND-GUIDED STERNOCLAVICULAR JOINT INJECTION

For the anterior out-of-plane approach to the SCJ, the patient is placed in the supine position with a few pillows under the upper back or the head of the bed elevated (**Fig. 3**A). Often, the clavicle at the SCJ lies superficial to the manubrium, creating a step-off that can be used as an anatomic landmark for locating the joint via palpation before transducer placement. A high-frequency (>10 MHz) linear-array transducer is placed long axis to the SCJ, placing the center of the joint in the center of the transducer (see **Fig. 3**A). Occasionally, in the setting of severe abnormality, passive shoulder motion may be used to dynamically move the clavicle relative to the manubrium to help identify the joint. Frequently, the joint will become more conspicuous by rotating the transducer slightly clockwise or counterclockwise. Color Doppler can be used to locate the common carotid artery, which lies deep to the SCJ and theoretically could be injured with needle misplacement (**Fig. 3**D). Once the SCJ is localized, a 25- to 27-gauge 25- to 38-mm needle is introduced via an out-of-plane anterior-to-posterior approach under direct USG to anesthetize the skin and needle track (**Fig. 3**C). Before injection, the clinician may rotate the transducer 90° to the long-axis view of the needle to assess depth and positioning (see **Fig. 3**D). Following proper placement within the SCJ, the syringe is exchanged; the needle position is sonographically reconfirmed, and the SCJ is injected with the desired amount of injectate (usually <1 mL) (Video 3). As with the ACJ injection described previously, care must be taken to avoid overdistension of the joint, and the goals of the injection must be considered because of the relatively small joint space.

GLENOHUMERAL JOINT

The glenohumeral joint (GHJ) is composed of a hyaline-covered spherical humeral head that articulates with the essentially flat hyaline-covered glenoid fossa.[1,53] The glenoid labrum, which is composed of fibrocartilage, increases the depth and width of the shallow glenoid fossa as well as GHJ stability.[54,55] There are several joint recesses associated with the GHJ, including the LHBBT sheath, the axillary recess, and the subscapular recess.[1,55,56]

Secondary to its increased range of motion and the relative incongruence between the glenoid fossa and the humeral head, the GHJ is prone to instability and abnormality.[57] The GHJ can be affected posttraumatically as a result of a dislocation or subluxation, with resultant labral injury, or a chronic RTC tear resulting in RTC arthropathy.[58–60] It can also be affected idiopathically as a result of osteoarthritis or from inflammatory causes, such as rheumatoid arthritis and adhesive capsulitis.[61,62] Adhesive capsulitis is a common disease process affecting up to 3% to 5% of the population and up to 20% of patients with diabetes.[61] Although the pathophysiology of the disease is not well understood, it is thought to result from an inflammatory condition in the GHJ capsule that eventually results in decreased capsular volume and glenohumeral range of motion.[61]

The GHJ is best visualized via a posterior acoustic window with a low-frequency (<10 MHz) curvilinear-array transducer placed short axis to the joint in the oblique axial plane.[1,7] Common US findings in patients with GHJ abnormality include cortical irregularities, joint effusions, labral tears, and osteophytes.[6,7]

In those patients that fail conservative measures, such as physical therapy and oral anti-inflammatory/analgesic medication, intra-articular GHJ injection may be indicated. Multiple publications have demonstrated the accuracy rate of PG GHJ injections, ranging between 50% and 96% in the cadaveric setting and 10% and 100% in the clinical setting.[12,63–68] The PG anterior approach was generally found to be more accurate than the posterior approach.[64,66–69] Both the anterior and the posterior USG approaches are well-described, with reported accuracy rates of 93% in a cadaveric model and 97% to 100% in a clinical setting.[65,70–73] There is emerging evidence in favor of the anterior approach at the RI for the treatment of adhesive capsulitis, with higher rates of capsular distension on magnetic resonance arthrography.[74,75]

AUTHORS' PREFERRED TECHNIQUE FOR ULTRASOUND-GUIDED GLENOHUMERAL JOINT INJECTION
Posterior Approach

For the posterior in-plane injection of the GHJ, the patient is positioned side-lying with the affected limb up, occasionally with a bolster under the arm for comfort (**Fig. 4**A). A low-frequency (<10 MHz) curvilinear-array transducer is placed long axis to the fibers of the infraspinatus in the anatomic axial oblique plane to the GHJ (see **Fig. 4**A). Occasionally in the setting of severe abnormality, passive shoulder motion may be used

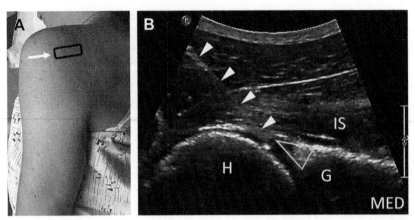

Fig. 4. US-guided posterior approach GHJ injection. (*A*) With the patient in the lateral decubitus position on the contralateral side, the transducer (*rectangle*) is placed just inferior to the spine of the scapula in an oblique axial plane to view the posterior GHJ. The needle trajectory (*arrow*) is via an in-plane posterolateral-to-anteromedial approach. (*B*) US image, with MED to the right, demonstrating a hyperechoic needle (*arrowheads*) deep to the glenoid (*triangle*) and within the posterior GHJ. See also Video 4.

to dynamically move the humerus relative to the glenoid to make the joint space more conspicuous. A 22- to 25-gauge 51- to 64-mm needle is introduced via an in-plane posterolateral approach under direct USG to anesthetize the skin and needle track into the GHJ (**Fig. 4**B). Care should be taken to avoid puncture of the glenoid labrum during the procedure, because this can be painful. After obtaining proper positioning, the syringe is exchanged; position is reconfirmed, and the GHJ is then injected with the desired amount of injectate (usually 4–5 mL) (Video 4).

In the case of adhesive capsulitis, higher volumes of injectate may be desired to produce capsular distension. Volumes of up to 20 mL have been reported without capsule rupture and with good clinical outcomes.[72,76–78] The practitioner may use a 2-needle technique in the case of adhesive capsulitis, with the first needle (usually 25-gauge 51-mm) being used to anesthetize the skin and needle track, and the second needle, introduced into the same insertion site, being 21-gauge or larger to allow for easier capsular distension. Care must also be taken to avoid overdistension of the joint, because this can result in debilitating postprocedure pain or capsular rupture.

Anterior Approach

For the anterior in-plane injection of the GHJ at the RI, the patient is positioned supine with the arm in external rotation to allow better visualization of the intra-articular LHBBT and RI. A high-frequency (>10 MHz) linear-array transducer is placed in the anatomic axial plane over the RI, short axis to the LHBBT (**Fig. 5**A). Following sterile preparation, a 25-gauge 51-mm needle is introduced via an in-plane lateral-to-medial fashion under direct USG to anesthetize the skin and needle track toward the RI. The needle is placed deep to the coracohumeral ligament and superficial to the LHBBT (**Fig. 5**B). After exchanging syringes, correct needle placement is sonographically reconfirmed and the GHJ is injected with the desired amount (usually 4–5 mL) (Video 5). Again, in the case of adhesive capsulitis, the practitioner may prefer a

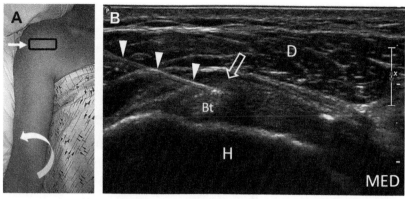

Fig. 5. US-guided anterior approach GHJ injection. (*A*) With the patient in the supine position and the arm externally rotated (*curved arrow*), the transducer (*rectangle*) is placed in the anatomic axial plane short axis to the LHBBT at the RI. The needle trajectory (*straight arrow*) is via an in-plane lateral-to-medial approach. (*B*) US image of an in-plane lateral-to-medial approach for needle placement (*arrowheads*) at the RI. Notice the needle is placed superficial to the Bt but deep to the coracohumeral ligament (*open arrow*) at the level of the RI. See also Video 5.

2-needle technique to facilitate easier capsular distension. With higher volumes of injectate used to produce capsular distension, the clinician should be aware of the same caveats as the posterior approach described above.

LONG HEAD OF THE BICEPS BRACHII TENDON

The LHBBT at the shoulder lies in the intertubercular groove created by the greater and lesser tuberosities of the humerus.[6,79] It is stabilized in the groove by the transverse humeral ligament, which is a combination of the coracohumeral ligament and the subscapularis and supraspinatus tendons.[79] At the RI, the LHBBT is further stabilized medially by the reflection pulley, which is an anatomic fibrous sling created by both the coracohumeral ligament and the superior glenohumeral ligament.[6,79] The LHBBT is surrounded by a tendon sheath, which communicates directly with the GHJ and extends approximately 3 to 4 cm distal to the intertubercular groove.[6,79]

The LHBBT is best visualized sonographically with a high-frequency (>10 MHz) linear-array transducer and should be evaluated in both the long and the short axis. US findings such as tendinopathy with tenosynovitis, dynamic biceps tendon subluxation or dislocation, and degenerative longitudinal split tearing are common abnormalities associated with a painful LHBBT (**Fig. 6**B).[80,81] Isolated tenosynovitis of the LHBBT is rare, and its incidence has been reported as low as 5%.[82] As previously mentioned, the LHBBT sheath communicates with the GHJ; therefore, tenosynovitis is found more commonly in association with RTC or GHJ abnormality.[7] In fact, rupture of the LHBBT rarely happens in isolation, occurring approximately 95% in association with RTC tears.[7] Therefore, the clinician should have a high suspicion for concomitant shoulder abnormality in the setting of LHBBT sheath effusion, rupture, or tenosynovitis.

For patients that have failed conservative management, injection of the biceps tendon sheath for both diagnostic and therapeutic purposes may be considered. There is a paucity of literature pertaining to the accuracy of PG LHBBT sheath injections. However, the accuracy of palpation of the LHBBT in the clinical setting has been

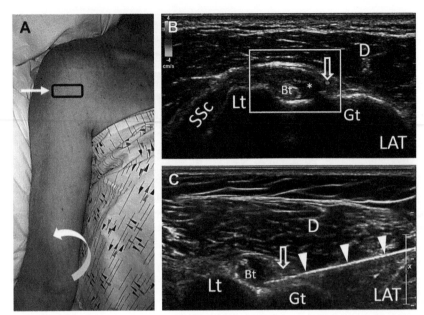

Fig. 6. US-guided LHBBT sheath injection. (*A*) With the patient in the supine position and the arm externally rotated (*curved arrow*), the transducer (*rectangle*) is placed in the anatomic axial plane short axis to the LHBBT at the bicipital groove. The needle trajectory (*straight arrow*) is via an in-plane lateral-to-medial approach. (*B*) Longitudinal split tearing of the Bt surrounded by a mixed heterogenic fluid (*asterix*) with hyperemia on low-flow color Doppler imaging (*within box*), consistent with tenosynovitis at the level of the bicipital groove. Note the anterior humeral circumflex artery (*open arrow*) on the LAT side of the tendon. (*C*) US image of an in-plane lateral-to-medial needle placement (*arrowheads*) deep to the LHBBT, while avoiding the anterior humeral circumflex artery (*open arrow*) at the level of the bicipital groove. See also Video 6.

shown to be difficult, with an accuracy range of 0% to 12%.[83] There is currently only one study evaluating the accuracy of PG versus USG injections into the LHBBT sheath, with reported accuracies of 27% and 87%, respectively.[84]

AUTHORS' PREFERRED TECHNIQUE FOR ULTRASOUND-GUIDED LONG HEAD BICEPS BRACHII TENDON SHEATH INJECTION

The anterior in-plane injection of the LHBBT sheath at the intertubercular groove is performed by first positioning the patient supine with the arm in external rotation to allow better visualization of the LHBBT in its anatomic short axis (**Fig. 6**A). A high-frequency (>10 MHz) linear-array transducer is placed in the anatomic axial plane over the intertubercular groove, short axis to the LHBBT. Color Doppler should be used to identify the ascending branch of the anterior humeral circumflex artery, which typically lies lateral to the LHBBT in the intertubercular groove (see **Fig. 6**B).[6] A 25-gauge 51-mm (or 25-gauge 38-mm depending on body habitus) needle is introduced via an in-plane lateral-to-medial fashion to anesthetize the skin and needle track toward the LHBBT sheath (**Fig. 6**C). The lesser tuberosity can be used as a bony backstop for the needle. Care should be taken to avoid the previously mentioned ascending branch of the anterior humeral circumflex artery (see **Fig. 6**B). Following correct placement, the syringe is exchanged; position is reconfirmed, and the sheath is injected with the desired amount of injectate (usually 3–5 mL) (Video 6).

CALCIFIC TENDINOPATHY/BURSOPATHY OF THE SHOULDER

Calcific tendinopathy of the shoulder is a common condition, occurring in up to 20% of all painful shoulders.[85,86] Women are predominantly affected more than men, with approximately 80% of cases involving the supraspinatus tendon, and a majority of cases associated with a nondegenerative RTC.[85] Pathophysiologically, the condition is thought to be related to mictrotraumatic factors and local decrease of oxygen concentration, resulting in fibrocartilaginous metaplasia and tendon necrosis followed by calcium hydroxyapatite deposition.[85,87] The resorption of the calcium deposition results in intratendinous edema and often acute, intense shoulder pain.[85,87] As with all RTC imaging, calcific tendinopathy of the RTC is best evaluated while using a high-frequency (>10 MHz) linear-array transducer. The calcific deposits can be classified as hard (hyperechoic, well-circumscribed, with posterior acoustic shadowing), soft (homogeneous hyperechoic with incomplete shadowing), or fluid (hyperechoic peripheral rim with hypoechoic/anechoic center and incomplete shadowing).[88,89] The latter two, which represent calcific deposits in the resorptive phase, are more amendable to lavage and aspiration (barbotage) (**Fig. 7**A, C).[86,88–90]

Many cases are self-limited (7–10 days) and require only noninvasive treatment.[6,85] It should also be noted that radiographically or sonographically identified calcifications of the RTC may be asymptomatic. Recalcitrant or extremely painful cases may require interventional management. Successful treatment with lithotripsy, arthroscopy, or open excision has been described.[90–93] USG calcific barbotage has been shown to be less invasive, more accessible, and associated with reduced postprocedural complications than arthroscopic or open procedures.[90] In a systemic review of 13 original articles involving 908 patients treated with USG calcific barbotage, with or without SASD bursa corticosteroid injection, subjects achieved an average of 55% improvement in pain and functional scores with a relatively low 10% complication rate.[90]

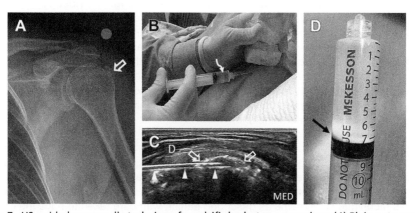

Fig. 7. US-guided one-needle technique for calcific barbotage procedure. (*A*) Plain anteroposterior external rotation view radiograph of a left shoulder demonstrating calcific deposit (*open arrow*) within the supraspinatus tendon. (*B*) For the in-plane lateral-to-medial approach, the patient is positioned supine, and the transducer is placed long axis to the supraspinatus and toggled to visualize the calcific deposit at its thickest point. Note the calcium being aspirated into the syringe (*curved arrow*). (*C*) US image of the hyperechoic needle (*arrowheads*) within the center of the borders of a calcific deposit (*open arrows*). (*D*) Calcium hydroxyapatite (*solid arrow*) within a syringe following calcific barbotage. See also Video 7.

AUTHORS' PREFERRED TECHNIQUE FOR ULTRASOUND-GUIDED PERCUTANEOUS CALCIFIC BARBOTAGE FOR CALCIFIC TENDINOPATHY
One-Needle Technique

For the in-plane, one-needle percutaneous USG calcific barbotage, the patient is positioned supine with several pillows under the upper back so that the needle and syringe can remain in a dependent position while the procedure is performed. Different positions may be required if a tendon other than the supraspinatus is affected. It is important to keep the needle and syringe in a dependent position if possible to aid with subsequent calcific deposit aspiration (**Fig. 7**B). A high-frequency (>10 MHz) linear-array transducer is placed in a position (usually anatomic coronal plane, long axis to the supraspinatus) that allows for optimal visualization of the calcific deposit (see **Fig. 7**C). A 25-gauge 51-mm needle is introduced via an in-plane lateral-to-medial fashion toward the calcific deposit. Care should be taken to avoid excessive fenestration of the calcific deposit before barbotage because this will affect the backpressure used to extract the deposit. Once adequate local anesthesia is obtained, this needle is withdrawn and an 18-gauge 51-mm needle is introduced down the anesthetized track. It is the authors' preference to fill the first 10 mL barbotage syringe with a mixture of 3 mL 2% lidocaine and 3 mL normal saline to provide further local anesthesia during the procedure.

As the clinician penetrates the calcium deposit, it is important to avoid puncture of the medial wall, because this will result in loss of backpressure and will often require conversion to a 2-needle technique (described later in this article). Once proper positioning in the center of the calcific deposit is sonographically confirmed, small aliquots of injectate are lavaged into the calcific deposit in a pumping fashion (see **Fig. 7**B, C). Note that there is usually a significant amount of resistance at the start of the procedure. Eventually, the resistance will decrease and the backpressure will pump the calcium hydroxyapatite back into the syringe. Once the syringe gets too cloudy to determine if additional calcium is being accumulated, it is exchanged for another 10-mL syringe that is filled with approximately 6 mL of normal saline, and the process is repeated until no additional calcium can be extracted (**Fig. 7**D, Video 7). Note this may take several syringes depending on the size of the calcific deposit. If the syringe gets clogged during the procedure, it can be unclogged using the technique described by Jelsing and colleagues.[94] First, the needle is withdrawn into the overlying deltoid muscle. Then, a 25-gauge 89-mm needle is threaded through the 18-gauge needle to dislodge the obstructive calcific debris. The barbotage procedure can then resume in the fashion described earlier. Following completion of the barbotage, the practitioner may wish to withdraw into the subacromial/subdeltoid bursa and inject corticosteroid, such as 40 mg triamcinolone.[90]

Two-Needle Technique

In cases in which backpressure is lost or a clinician is unable to barbotage the calcium with a 1-needle technique, a 2-needle technique may be used. The patient positioning for this technique is the same as described earlier, with care taken to have the open aspiration needle in a dependent position (**Fig. 8**A, B). A 25-gauge 51-mm needle is introduced via an in-plane lateral-to-medial approach under direct USG toward the calcific deposit. Once adequate anesthesia is obtained, this needle is withdrawn, and an 18-gauge 51-mm needle is introduced down the anesthetized track into the calcific deposit. Following this, another 25-gauge 51-mm needle is introduced in a dependent position to the already introduced 18-gauge needle. Once adequate anesthesia is obtained, this needle is then withdrawn and a second 18-gauge 51 mm

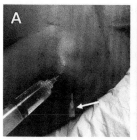
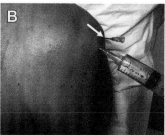
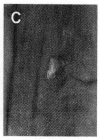

Fig. 8. US-guided 2-needle technique for calcific barbotage procedure. (*A, B*) Anterior and lateral views of needle positioning for 2-needle technique for calcific barbotage procedure. Note the dependent position of the open needle (*arrow*). (*C*) Irrigated calcium hydroxyapatite on a sterile blue towel.

needle is introduced down the anesthetized track under direct USG (see **Fig. 8**A, B). The syringe is removed, and this needle is left open to drain. The transducer is then repositioned long axis to the first needle, and the calcific deposition is irrigated with several syringes of normal saline, while allowing fluid and calcium to be aspirated out of the open syringe (**Fig. 8**C). Following completion of the barbotage, the second introduced needle is withdrawn completely. The clinician may wish to reposition the first needle into the SASD bursa and inject corticosteroid, such as 40 mg of triamcinolone.[90]

SUMMARY

In conclusion, multiple pathologic conditions of the shoulder can be treated with USG interventions. With its accessibility, portability, lack of contraindications, and increased accuracy, USG procedures have several potential advantages over PG or fluoroscopically guided procedures. Therefore, clinicians should strongly consider using USG for minimally invasive procedures of the shoulder.

SUPPLEMENTARY DATA

Supplementary data related to this article can be found at http://dx.doi.org/10.1016/j.pmr.2016.04.001.

REFERENCES

1. Finnoff J, Smith J, Peck E. Ultrasonography of the shoulder. Phys Med Rehabil Clin N Am 2010;21(3):481–507.
2. Smith J, Finnoff J. Diagnostic and interventional musculoskeletal ultrasound: part 2. Clinical applications. PM R 2009;1(2):162–77.
3. Smith J, Finnoff J. Diagnostic and interventional musculoskeletal ultrasound: part 1. PM R 2009;1(1):64–75.
4. Hall M. The accuracy and efficacy of palpation versus image-guided peripheral injections in sports medicine. Curr Sports Med Rep 2013;12(5):296–303.
5. Finnoff J, Hall M, Adams E, et al. American Medical Society for Sports Medicine (AMSSM) position statement: interventional musculoskeletal ultrasound in sports medicine. Br J Sports Med 2015;49(3):145–50.
6. Bianchi S. Ultrasound of the musculoskeletal system. 1st edition. Verlag (Germany): Springer; 2007.

7. Jacobson J. Fundamentals of musculoskeletal ultrasound. 2nd edition. Philadelphia: Saunders; 2013.

8. Draghi F, Scudeller L, Draghi AG, et al. Prevalence of subacromial-subdeltoid bursitis in shoulder pain: an ultrasonographic study. J Ultrasound 2015;18(2): 151–8.

9. Gasparre G, Fusaro I, Galletti S, et al. Effectiveness of ultrasound-guided injections combined with shoulder exercises in the treatment of subacromial adhesive bursitis. Musculoskelet Surg 2012;96(Suppl 1):S57–61.

10. Chen MJ, Lew HL, Hsu TC, et al. Ultrasound-guided shoulder injections in the treatment of subacromial bursitis. Am J Phys Med Rehabil 2006;85(1):31–5.

11. Cadogan A, Laslett M, Hing W, et al. Clinical predictors of a positive response to guided diagnostic block into the subacromial bursa. J Rehabil Med 2012;44(10): 877–84.

12. Eustace J, Brophy D, Gibney R, et al. Comparison of the accuracy of steroid placement with clinical outcome in patients with shoulder symptoms. Ann Rheum Dis 1997;56(1):59–63.

13. Kang M, Rizio L, Prybicien M, et al. The accuracy of subacromial corticosteroid injections: a comparison of multiple methods. J Shoulder Elbow Surg 2008; 17(Suppl 1):61S–6S.

14. Mathews P, Glousman R. Accuracy of subacromial injection: anterolateral versus posterior approach. J Shoulder Elbow Surg 2005;14(2):145–8.

15. Partington P, Broome G. Diagnostic injection around the shoulder: hit and miss? A cadaveric study of injection accuracy. J Shoulder Elbow Surg 1998;7(2):147–50.

16. Yamakado K. The targeting accuracy of subacromial injection to the shoulder: an arthrographic evaluation. Arthroscopy 2002;18(8):887–91.

17. Dogu B, Yucel S, Sag S, et al. Blind or ultrasound-guided corticosteroid injections and short-term response in subacromial impingement syndrome: a randomized, double-blind, prospective study. Am J Phys Med Rehabil 2012;91(8):658–65.

18. Rutten M, Maresch B, Jager G, et al. Injection of the subacromial-subdeltoid bursa: blind or ultrasound-guided? Acta Orthop 2007;78(2):254–7.

19. Saccomanno MF, DE Ieso C, Milano G. Acromioclavicular joint instability: anatomy, biomechanics and evaluation. Joints 2014;2(2):87–92.

20. Mall N, Foley E, Chalmers P, et al. Degenerative joint disease of the acromioclavicular joint: a review. Am J Sports Med 2013;41(11):2684–92.

21. Shubin Stein B, Ahmad C, Pfaff C, et al. A comparison of magnetic resonance imaging findings of the acromioclavicular joint in symptomatic versus asymptomatic patients. J Shoulder Elbow Surg 2006;15(1):56–9.

22. Stein B, Wiater J, Pfaff H, et al. Detection of acromioclavicular joint pathology in asymptomatic shoulders with magnetic resonance imaging. J Shoulder Elbow Surg 2001;10(3):204–8.

23. Chronopoulos E, Kim T, Park H, et al. Diagnostic value of physical tests for isolated chronic acromioclavicular lesions. Am J Sports Med 2004;32(3):655–61.

24. Walton J, Mahajan S, Paxinos A, et al. Diagnostic values of tests for acromioclavicular joint pain. J Bone Joint Surg Am 2004;86-A(4):807–12.

25. Alasaarela E, Tervonen O, Takalo R, et al. Ultrasound evaluation of the acromioclavicular joint. J Rheumatol 1997;24(10):1959–63.

26. Tallia A, Cardone D. Diagnostic and therapeutic injection of the shoulder region. Am Fam Physician 2003;67(6):1271–8.

27. Gerber C, Galantay R, Hersche O. The pattern of pain produced by irritation of the acromioclavicular joint and the subacromial space. J Shoulder Elbow Surg 1998;7(4):352–5.

28. Borbas P, Kraus T, Clement H, et al. The influence of ultrasound guidance in the rate of success of acromioclavicular joint injection: an experimental study on human cadavers. J Shoulder Elbow Surg 2012;21(12):1694–7.
29. Peck E, Lai J, Pawlina W, et al. Accuracy of ultrasound-guided versus palpation-guided acromioclavicular joint injections: a cadaveric study. PM R 2010;2(9): 817–21.
30. Sabeti-Aschraf M, Lemmerhofer B, Lang S, et al. Ultrasound guidance improves the accuracy of the acromioclavicular joint infiltration: a prospective randomized study. Knee Surg Sports Traumatol Arthrosc 2011;19(2):292–5.
31. Wasserman B, Pettrone S, Jazrawi L, et al. Accuracy of acromioclavicular joint injections. Am J Sports Med 2013;41(1):149–52.
32. Sabeti-Aschraf M, Ochsner A, Schueller-Weidekamm C, et al. The infiltration of the AC joint performed by one specialist: ultrasound versus palpation a prospective randomized pilot study. Eur J Radiol 2010;75(1):e37–40.
33. Tubbs R, Loukas M, Slappey J, et al. Surgical and clinical anatomy of the interclavicular ligament. Surg Radiol Anat 2007;29(5):357–60.
34. van Tongel A, MacDonald P, Leiter J, et al. A cadaveric study of the structural anatomy of the sternoclavicular joint. Clin Anat 2012;25(7):903–10.
35. Barbaix E, Lapierre M, Van Roy P, et al. The sternoclavicular joint: variants of the discus articularis. Clin Biomech (Bristol, Avon) 2000;15(Suppl 1):S3–7.
36. Bearn J. Direct observations on the function of the capsule of the sternoclavicular joint in clavicular support. J Anat 1967;101(Pt 1):159–70.
37. Rodríguez-Henríquez P, Solano C, Peña A, et al. Sternoclavicular joint involvement in rheumatoid arthritis: clinical and ultrasound findings of a neglected joint. Arthritis Care Res (Hoboken) 2013;65(7):1177–82.
38. Antohe J, Delvecchio B, Harrington T. An unusual presentation of acute calcium pyrophosphate dihydrate arthropathy of the sternoclavicular joint in a patient with systemic lupus erythematosus. J Clin Rheumatol 2012;18(3):162.
39. Klein M, Spreitzer A, Miro P, et al. MR imaging of the abnormal sternoclavicular joint–a pictorial essay. Clin Imaging 1997;21(2):138–43.
40. Kier R, Wain S, Apple J, et al. Osteoarthritis of the sternoclavicular joint. Radiographic features and pathologic correlation. Invest Radiol 1986;21(3):227–33.
41. Sadr B, Swann M. Spontaneous dislocation of the sterno-clavicular joint. Acta Orthop Scand 1979;50(3):269–74.
42. Jung J, Molinger M, Kohn D, et al. Intra-articular glucocorticosteroid injection into sternocostoclavicular joints in patients with SAPHO syndrome. Semin Arthritis Rheum 2012;42(3):266–70.
43. Levy M, Goldberg I, Fischel R, et al. Friedrich's disease: aseptic necrosis of the sternal end of the clavicle. J Bone Joint Surg Br 1981;63(4):539–41.
44. Hassett G, Barnsley L. Pain referral from the sternoclavicular joint: a study in normal volunteers. Rheumatology (Oxford) 2001;40(8):859–62.
45. Brossmann J, Stäbler A, Preidler K, et al. Sternoclavicular joint: MR imaging–anatomic correlation. Radiology 1996;198(1):193–8.
46. Wisniewski S, Smith J. Synovitis of the sternoclavicular joint: the role of ultrasound. Am J Phys Med Rehabil 2007;86(4):322–3.
47. Johnson M, Jacobson J, Fessell D, et al. The sternoclavicular joint: can imaging differentiate infection from degenerative change? Skeletal Radiol 2010;39(6): 551–8.
48. Galla R, Basava V, Conermann T, et al. Sternoclavicular steroid injection for treatment of pain in a patient with osteitis condensans of the clavicle. Pain Physician 2009;12(6):987–90.

49. Peterson C, Saupe N, Buck F, et al. CT-guided sternoclavicular joint injections: description of the procedure, reliability of imaging diagnosis, and short-term patient responses. AJR Am J Roentgenol 2010;195(6):435–9.

50. Weinberg A, Pichler W, Grechenig S, et al. Frequency of successful intra-articular puncture of the sternoclavicular joint: a cadaver study. Scand J Rheumatol 2009; 38(5):396–8.

51. Taneja A, Bierry G, Simeone F, et al. Diagnostic yield of CT-guided sampling in suspected sternoclavicular joint infection. Skeletal Radiol 2013;42(4):479–85.

52. Pourcho A, Sellon J, Smith J. Sonographically guided sternoclavicular joint injection: description of technique and validation. J Ultrasound Med 2015;34(2): 325–31.

53. Culham E, Peat M. Functional anatomy of the shoulder complex. J Orthop Sports Phys Ther 1993;18(1):342–50.

54. Kwak SM, Brown RR, Resnick D, et al. Anatomy, anatomic variations, and pathology of the 11- to 3-o'clock position of the glenoid labrum: findings on MR arthrography and anatomic sections. AJR Am J Roentgenol 1998;171(1):235–8.

55. Cooper DE, Arnoczky SP, O'Brien SJ, et al. Anatomy, histology, and vascularity of the glenoid labrum. An anatomical study. J Bone Joint Surg Am 1992;74(1): 46–52.

56. De Maeseneer M, Van Roy P, Shahabpour M. Normal MR imaging anatomy of the rotator cuff tendons, glenoid fossa, labrum, and ligaments of the shoulder. Radiol Clin North Am 2006;44(4):479–87.

57. Longo UG, Rizzello G, Loppini M, et al. Multidirectional instability of the shoulder: a systematic review. Arthroscopy 2015;31(12):2431–43.

58. Nam D, Maak T, Raphael B, et al. Rotator cuff tear arthropathy: evaluation, diagnosis, and treatment: AAOS exhibit selection. J Bone Joint Surg Am 2012;94(6): E34.

59. Clavert P. Glenoid labrum pathology. Orthop Traumatol Surg Res 2015;101(Suppl 1):S19–24.

60. Thangarajah T, Lambert S. Management of the unstable shoulder. BMJ 2015;350: H2537.

61. Robinson C, Seah K, Chee Y, et al. Frozen shoulder. J Bone Joint Surg Br 2012; 94(1):1–9.

62. Izquierdo R, Voloshin I, Edwards S, et al. Treatment of glenohumeral osteoarthritis. J Am Acad Orthop Surg 2010;18(6):375–82.

63. Catalano O, Manfredi R, Vanzulli A, et al. MR arthrography of the glenohumeral joint: modified posterior approach without imaging guidance. Radiology 2007; 242(2):550–4.

64. DeMouy EH, Menendez CV Jr, Bodin CJ. Palpation-directed (non-fluoroscopically guided) saline-enhanced MR arthrography of the shoulder. AJR Am J Roentgenol 1997;169(1):229–31.

65. Choudur HN, Ellins ML. Ultrasound-guided gadolinium joint injections for magnetic resonance arthrography. J Clin Ultrasound 2011;39(1):6–11.

66. Naredo E, Cabero F, Beneyto P, et al. A randomized comparative study of short term response to blind injection versus sonographic-guided injection of local corticosteroids in patients with painful shoulder. J Rheumatol 2004;31(2):308–14.

67. Sethi PM, El Attrache N. Accuracy of intra-articular injection of the glenohumeral joint: a cadaveric study. Orthopedics 2006;29(2):149–52.

68. Sethi PM, Kingston S, Elattrache N. Accuracy of anterior intra-articular injection of the glenohumeral joint. Arthroscopy 2005;21(1):77–80.

69. Tobola A, Cook C, Cassas KJ, et al. Accuracy of glenohumeral joint injections: comparing approach and experience of provider. J Shoulder Elbow Surg 2011; 20(7):1147–54.
70. Patel DN, Nayyar S, Hasan S, et al. Comparison of ultrasound-guided versus blind glenohumeral injections: a cadaveric study. J Shoulder Elbow Surg 2012; 21(12):1664–8.
71. Gokalp G, Dusak A, Yazici Z. Efficacy of ultrasonography-guided shoulder MR arthrography using a posterior approach. Skeletal Radiol 2010;39(6):575–9.
72. Souza PM, Aguiar RO, Marchiori E, et al. Arthrography of the shoulder: a modified ultrasound guided technique of joint injection at the rotator interval. Eur J Radiol 2010;74(3):e29–32.
73. Zwar RB, Read JW, Noakes JB. Sonographically guided glenohumeral joint injection. AJR Am J Roentgenol 2004;183(1):48–50.
74. Prestgaard T, Wormgoor ME, Haugen S, et al. Ultrasound-guided intra-articular and rotator interval corticosteroid injections in adhesive capsulitis of the shoulder: a double-blind, sham-controlled randomized study. Pain 2015;156(9):1683–91.
75. Ogul H, Bayraktutan U, Ozgokce M, et al. Ultrasound-guided shoulder MR arthrography: comparison of rotator interval and posterior approach. Clin Imaging 2014;38(1):11–7.
76. Ahn JK, Kim J, Lee SJ, et al. Effects of ultrasound-guided intra-articular ketorolac injection with capsular distension. J Back Musculoskelet Rehabil 2015;28(3): 497–503.
77. Park KD, Nam HS, Lee JK, et al. Treatment effects of ultrasound-guided capsular distension with hyaluronic acid in adhesive capsulitis of the shoulder. Arch Phys Med Rehabil 2013;94(2):264–70.
78. Jacobs LG, Smith MG, Khan SA, et al. Manipulation or intra-articular steroids in the management of adhesive capsulitis of the shoulder? A prospective randomized trial. J Shoulder Elbow Surg 2009;18(3):348–53.
79. Elser F, Braun S, Dewing CB, et al. Anatomy, function, injuries, and treatment of the long head of the biceps brachii tendon. Arthroscopy 2011;27(4):581–92.
80. Walch G, Nove-Josserand L, Boileau P, et al. Subluxations and dislocations of the tendon of the long head of the biceps. J Shoulder Elbow Surg 1998;7(2):100–8.
81. Wu PT, Jou IM, Yang CC, et al. The severity of the long head biceps tendinopathy in patients with chronic rotator cuff tears: macroscopic versus microscopic results. J Shoulder Elbow Surg 2014;23(8):1099–106.
82. Patton WC, McCluskey GM 3rd. Biceps tendinitis and subluxation. Clin Sports Med 2001;20(3):505–29.
83. Gazzillo GP, Finnoff JT, Hall MM, et al. Accuracy of palpating the long head of the biceps tendon: an ultrasonographic study. PM R 2011;3(11):1035–40.
84. Hashiuchi T, Sakurai G, Morimoto M, et al. Accuracy of the biceps tendon sheath injection: ultrasound-guided or unguided injection? A randomized controlled trial. J Shoulder Elbow Surg 2011;20(7):1069–73.
85. Speed CA, Hazleman BL. Calcific tendinitis of the shoulder. N Engl J Med 1999; 340(20):1582–4.
86. Serafini G, Sconfienza L, Lacelli F, et al. Rotator cuff calcific tendonitis: short-term and 10-year outcomes after two-needle us-guided percutaneous treatment–non-randomized controlled trial. Radiology 2009;252(1):157–64.
87. De Carli A, Pulcinelli F, Rose GD, et al. Calcific tendinitis of the shoulder. Joints 2014;2(3):130–6.

88. Farin PU, Rasanen H, Jaroma H, et al. Rotator cuff calcifications: treatment with ultrasound-guided percutaneous needle aspiration and lavage. Skeletal Radiol 1996;25(6):551–4.

89. Sconfienza L, Bandirali M, Serafini G, et al. Rotator cuff calcific tendinitis: does warm saline solution improve the short-term outcome of double-needle US-guided treatment? Radiology 2012;262(2):560–6.

90. Gatt DL, Charalambous CP. Ultrasound-guided barbotage for calcific tendonitis of the shoulder: a systematic review including 908 patients. Arthroscopy 2014; 30(9):1166–72.

91. Vavken P, Holinka J, Rompe JD, et al. Focused extracorporeal shock wave therapy in calcifying tendinitis of the shoulder: a meta-analysis. Sports Health 2009; 1(2):137–44.

92. Maier D, Jaeger M, Izadpanah K, et al. Arthroscopic treatment of calcific tendinitis of the shoulder. Am J Sports Med 2012;40(7):NP12–13 [author reply: NP13].

93. Jerosch J, Strauss JM, Schmiel S. Arthroscopic treatment of calcific tendinitis of the shoulder. J Shoulder Elbow Surg 1998;7(1):30–7.

94. Jelsing E, Maida E, Smith J. A simple technique to restore needle patency during percutaneous lavage and aspiration of calcific rotator cuff tendinopathy. PM R 2013;5(3):242–4.

Ultrasound-Guided Elbow Procedures

Walter I. Sussman, DO[a,b], Christopher J. Williams, MD[a], Ken Mautner, MD[a,b],*

KEYWORDS

- Epicondylitis • Epicondylosis • Tendinopathy • Sonography • Tendinopathy
- Ultrasound • Ultrasound-guided injection

KEY POINTS

- Ultrasound is a useful modality for the evaluation of musculoskeletal elbow disorders and for the guidance of procedures in the elbow region.
- Current evidence shows that ultrasound-guided injections in the elbow region have superior accuracy to anatomic landmark–guided injections in the elbow region, although larger, higher-quality evidence is needed.
- Lateral epicondylosis is a common cause of elbow disorder, and ultrasound guidance is increasingly useful for the effective and precise delivery of novel treatments into this tendon.

INTRODUCTION

The elbow is a synovial joint with 3 articulations between the humerus, radius, and ulna (ulnohumeral, radiocapitellar, and proximal radioulnar joints) and 2 planes of motion (flexion/extension and pronation/supination). Functioning as a modified hinge joint, the elbow assists in positioning the hand in space, providing a powerful grasp and serving as a fulcrum for the forearm.[1–3] The joint must be flexible enough to accommodate these complex movements and stable enough to transmit forces from the hand through the shoulder. The interlocking bony anatomy of the elbow makes it inherently stable, but the capsuloligamentous restraints and elbow musculature also play a role.[4] Although high-resolution ultrasound (US) can help clinicians easily visualize key anatomic structures, understanding the complex anatomy and biomechanics of the elbow is essential to the successful diagnosis and treatment of common disorders.

Musculoskeletal clinicians frequently perform periarticular and intra-articular injections to manage elbow disorders. Historically, most procedures done around the elbow have been done using anatomic landmark guidance without live imaging;

Conflicts of Interest: The authors have no conflicts of interest to report.
[a] Department of Physical Medicine and Rehabilitation, Emory University, 1441 Clifton Road, NE Atlanta, GA 30322, USA; [b] Department of Orthopaedic Surgery, Emory University, Atlanta, GA, USA
* Corresponding author. Sports Medicine Center, 59 Executive Park South, Atlanta, GA 30329.
E-mail address: kmautne@emory.edu

Phys Med Rehabil Clin N Am 27 (2016) 573–587
http://dx.doi.org/10.1016/j.pmr.2016.04.002
1047-9651/16/$ – see front matter © 2016 Elsevier Inc. All rights reserved.

however, a recent review and position statement by the American Medical Society for Sports Medicine[5] found that US-guided injections (USGI) had improved accuracy, efficacy, and cost-effectiveness compared with landmark-guided injections (LMGI) for large joints (eg, knees and shoulders). Few studies have assessed the accuracy of USGI for the elbow,[6–10] and a review of the current literature found only 3 head-to-head studies comparing LMGI with USGI around the elbow,[6,7,9] and all 3 examined only intra-articular injections.

Given that the success of an injection often depends on placing the needle within the intended target, US is a safe, accessible, and inexpensive tool to ensure accurate needle placement. This article reviews common musculoskeletal disorders of the elbow (**Table 1**) that can be evaluated with US, reviews the literature on USGI of the elbow, and describes the senior author's preferred approach to the most common injections.

LATERAL EVALUATION

On US, the common extensor tendon normally has a hyperechoic fibrillar appearance. Changes in tendon echogenicity (generally increased hypoechogenicity), thickening of the tendon, cortical irregularity, intratendinous calcification, and/or tendon hyperemia signify degenerative changes and are seen with lateral epicondylosis.[11] Deep to the common extensor tendon lies the radial (lateral) collateral ligament, which typically occupies approximately 50% of footprint at the lateral epicondyle, and should also be assessed with the lateral evaluation.[12]

Lateral Epicondylosis

First described in 1882,[13] lateral epicondylosis is the most common cause of lateral elbow pain.[14] Pathologic changes typically occur within the deep-anterior fibers of the common extensor tendon at its origin on the lateral epicondyle.[11] Therapeutic injections have long been a cornerstone of management for lateral epicondylosis. Once thought to be an inflammatory process, glucocorticoid injections were used as early as the 1950s to help treat local inflammation in this condition.[15] Lateral epicondylosis is now recognized as a degenerative process, but despite this shift in understanding, corticosteroids remain the most common injectate studied and the most common substance injected.[16] Numerous randomized controlled trials have compared LMGI with corticosteroids versus local anesthetics,[17–19] saline injections,[20] prolotherapy,[21] physical therapy,[22–24] and observation (the wait-and-see approach).[23,25] Many of these studies showed short-term symptomatic relief; however, these benefits are often not sustained. Long-term studies have shown that corticosteroid injections are no more beneficial than observation alone, and may even have an inferior outcome with higher recurrence rates at 1 year.[23,25]

Studies of USGI of corticosteroid for lateral epicondylosis are limited. McShane and colleagues[26] presented 2 case series of patients with chronic lateral epicondylosis treated with US-guided percutaneous needle tenotomy.[27] In the 2006 study, subjects underwent fenestration of the common extensor tendon followed by an injection of corticosteroid and bupivacaine.[26] In a subsequent 2008 study, McShane and colleagues[27] repeated the same protocol, but without the corticosteroid and found superior results. The investigators concluded that corticosteroid injections are not a necessary component of the procedure.[27] In a 2013 randomized controlled trial, Krogh and colleagues[20] compared USGI with corticosteroids, platelet-rich plasma (PRP) and saline injections. Sixty patients were enrolled, with 20 in each treatment arm, and there was no significant difference in pain reduction between the 3 groups at 3 months. One

Table 1 Anatomic structures[a] and corresponding selected disorders of the elbow		
Anterior	Joint space, anterior coronoid recess	Effusion, synovial hypertrophy, loose bodies
	Humeroradial/humeroulnar joint, coronoid and radial fossae	Integrity of the articular cartilage and cortical bone, fracture
	Annular recess and neck of the radius	Effusion, synovial hypertrophy, loose bodies, dynamic assessment of radial head in supination and pronation for radial head subluxation
	Distal biceps tendon	Full-thickness or partial-thickness tears, tendinosis, bicipitoradial bursitis
	Brachialis muscle	—
	Median nerve	Entrapment at level of distal humerus (ligament of Struthers), antecubital region (pronator teres), atrophy of distal muscles
	Radial nerve	Supinator syndrome or radial tunnel syndrome (hypoechoic swelling of nerve at entry of Arcade of Fröhse)
	Radial and brachial vessels	—
Lateral	Lateral epicondyle, common extensor tendon, proximal attachments of the extensor carpi radialis longus and brachioradialis	Epicondylosis, adjacent bone irregularity, full-thickness or partial-thickness tear (former is uncommon)
	Radial collateral ligament	Ligament tear
Medial	Medial epicondyle/common flexor tendon	Epicondylosis, adjacent bone irregularity
	Ulnar collateral ligament	Full-thickness or partial-thickness tear, laxity on dynamic examination
	Ulnar nerve in cubital tunnel	Nerve entrapment (hypoechoic swelling of ulnar nerve), dynamic examination with elbow flexion and extension to assess for subluxation, snapping triceps syndrome, anconeus epitrochlearis muscle
Posterior	Posterior joint space (olecranon recess) and olecranon process	Effusion with elevation of the hyperechoic fat pad, synovial hypertrophy, loose bodies, fracture
	Distal triceps tendon	Full-thickness or partial-thickness tears, distal avulsion, tendinosis
	Olecranon bursa	Bursitis, synovial hypertrophy/proliferation
	Distal biceps tendon insertion	Dynamic evaluation of insertion at radial tuberosity with pronation and supination

[a] Anatomic structures as outlined in the American Institute of Ultrasound in Medicine practice parameters for the US examination of the elbow.[68]

significant limitation of this study was that, despite a predetermined 12-month study interval, the 6-month and 12-month outcomes were not reported because of a significant number of patients being lost to follow-up, and the maximum benefits from a PRP injection may not be realized until 6 months after the injection.[28]

Once the gold standard for the treatment of lateral epicondylosis, glucocorticoid injections are now considered to have a deleterious effect on this condition, and a growing number of novel injection therapies for lateral epicondylosis have been reported in the literature. Randomized studies have examined the role of botulinum toxin,[29,30] prolotherapy,[21,31,32] and sclerosing solutions.[33–35] Despite botulinum toxin being the second most studied injectate in randomized controlled trials,[16] no studies have examined USGI with botulinum toxin for lateral epicondylosis. A growing body of literature has also examined autologous whole-blood injections,[36,37] PRP,[20,28,38,39] autologous stem cell therapy,[40] and percutaneous needle tenotomy[26,27,41] to augment the natural healing process. These procedures are discussed in more detail elsewhere in this issue.

US guidance has been used in a few of these studies using novel injectate (**Table 2**). In 2013, Rabago and colleagues[31] presented a prospective randomized controlled trial of USGI of prolotherapy with 3 treatment arms: (1) 20% dextrose solution (PrT-D), (2) dextrose-morrhuate sodium (PrT-DM) solution, and (3) observation. The 2 prolotherapy groups showed improvement in Patient-rated Tennis Elbow Evaluation composite scores at both 16 and 32 weeks' follow-up compared with the observation group. The PrT-D group had less pain and improved grip strength compared with the other groups.[31] In 2006, Zeisig and colleagues[33] presented a pilot study of USGI of polidocanol, a local anesthetic and sclerosant. Although the pilot study showed a significant improvement in pain and grip strength at 8 months, a larger prospective randomized controlled study failed to reproduce these results at 3-month, 12-month,[34] or 24-month follow-up,[35] and a network meta-analysis found no significant difference between polidocanol and placebo.[16]

Sonographic Needle Placement

US findings of lateral epicondylosis have been well documented,[11] but no studies have compared USGI versus LMGI for the treatment of this condition. Depending on the injectate, the precise needle target around the common extensor tendon may vary. For example, corticosteroid injections have traditionally targeted the peritendinous region superficial to the common extensor tendon. However, with the novel treatments described earlier (eg, percutaneous needle fenestration, orthobiologics) the needle should be directed into areas of abnormality within the tendon.

The patient is positioned in a seated or supine position with the elbow flexed to approximately 90°, forearm prone, and the lateral aspect of the elbow facing the clinician. The US transducer is positioned in long axis to the common extensor tendon, the needle oriented in plane to the transducer, and the needle is advanced in a distal to proximal direction (**Fig. 1**). The length of the needle is typically 25 to 38 mm given the superficial nature of the common extensor tendon; the needle may vary from 18 to 25 gauge depending on the indication and goals of the procedure. Injectate volume likewise may vary but is typically 2 to 3 mL.

MEDIAL EVALUATION

The common flexor tendon originates from the medial epicondyle, and is shorter and broader than the common extensor tendon. The normal tendon appears as a hyperechoic fibrillary structure and pathologic changes are characterized by degenerative changes, similar to those with lateral epicondylosis described earlier.[42] The medial evaluation should also include examination of the anterior band of the ulnar (medial) collateral ligament (UCL), which is the major stabilizer of valgus stress at the elbow. Normally, the anterior band of the UCL appears as a fibrillar, hyperechoic, fanlike structure traversing from the medial epicondyle to its insertion on the sublime tubercle

Table 2
Summary of literature on USGI for elbow disorders and level of evidence

	Procedure	Number of Subjects	Duration of Follow-up (wk)	Study Design	Level of Evidence[a]
Lateral Epicondylosis					
Corticosteroids					
McShane et al,[26] 2006	PNT + CSI	58	121 (range 73–191)	Cohort	III
McShane et al,[27] 2008	PNT	52	88 (range 28–152)	Cohort	III
Prolotherapy					
Rabago et al,[31] 2013	PRT-D vs PRT-DM vs observation	26 (32 elbows)	32	RCT	II
Sclerosing Therapy					
Zeisig et al,[33] 2006	Polidocanol	11 (13 elbows)	35	Cohort	III
Zeisig et al,[34] 2008	Polidocanol	32 (36 elbows)	52	Cohort	III
Zeisig et al,[35] 2010	Polidocanol	25 (28 elbows)	104	Cohort	III
Orthobiologics					
Connell et al,[36] 2006	Autologous blood + PNT	35	26	Cohort	III
Connell et al,[40] 2009	Autologous dermal fibroblast	12	26	Cohort	III
Stenhouse et al,[41] 2013	Autologous conditioned plasma + PNT vs PNT	28	26	RCT	II
Krogh et al,[20] 2013	PRP vs CSI vs saline (PNT)	60	13	RCT	II[b]
Medial Epicondylosis					
Suresh et al,[47] 2006	Autologous blood + PNT	20	44	Cohort	III
Ulnar Collateral Ligament Disorders					
Podesta et al,[50] 2013	PRP	34	70 (range 11–117)	Cohort	III
Distal Biceps Disorders					
Sanli et al,[58] 2014	Intratendon PRP	12	47 (range 36–52)	Cohort	III
Barker et al,[59] 2015	Intratendon PRP	6	16.3 (range 12–30)	Cohort	III
Mautner et al,[57] 2015	Intratendon PRP	1	18	Case report	IV

Abbreviations: CSI, corticosteroid injection; PNT, percutaneous needle tenotomy; PRP, platelet-rich plasma; PRT-D, prolotherapy with 20% dextrose solution; PRT-DM, prolotherapy with dextrose-morrhuate sodium; RCT, randomized controlled trial.
 [a] Level of evidence was assigned through collaboration between 2 of the authors according to guidelines set forth by Wright.[69]
 [b] Less than 80% follow-up for predetermined study interval.

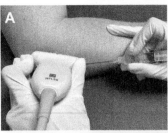
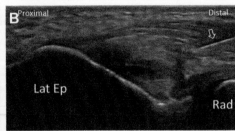
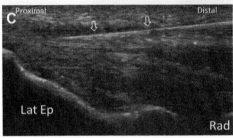

Fig. 1. Technique for US-guided percutaneous injection of the common extensor tendon with a longitudinal, in-plane approach (*A*). US images depicting an intratendinous injection (*B*) with the needle (*open arrows*) approaching the hypoechoic defect, and peritendinous (*C*) needle placement. The lateral epicondyle (Lat Ep) and proximal radius (Rad) serve as bony acoustic landmarks.

of the coronoid process on the ulna. Dynamic assessment of the UCL can be performed by placing the elbow under valgus stress with the elbow in slight flexion to disengage the olecranon. Complete tears result in discontinuity of the ligament and widening of the ulnohumeral joint with greater than a 0.5-mm difference between rest and stress, whereas partial tears can result in thickening of the ligament with internal disruption.[43] The ulnar nerve can also be assessed at the elbow, and should be dynamically examined for signs of entrapment or subluxation.

Medial Epicondylosis

Medial epicondylosis is not as common as its lateral counterpart, which is diagnosed 7 to 10 times more often.[44] Although a growing body of literature has explored different types of therapeutic injections for chronic lateral epicondylosis, the literature is limited for medial epicondylosis. Corticosteroids are the only injectate that has been studied in prospective randomized controlled trials, and neither of these 2 studies used US guidance.[45,46] Similar to lateral epicondylosis, subjects showed a short-term benefit, but had no sustained benefit at 3 months or 1 year.[46]

US guidance has only been used in 1 prospective cohort study for chronic medial epicondylosis.[47] In 2006, Suresh and colleagues[47] presented 20 subjects with US-guided needle fenestration followed by an injection of autologous blood (2 mL) into the site of maximum tendon injury. A second autologous blood injection, also 2 mL, was performed at 4 weeks' follow-up. Three of the 20 patients failed to improve following the procedure, but at the 10-month follow-up interval the remaining 17 patients had improvement in Visual Analog Scale pain scores and Nirschl elbow scores.

Sonographic Needle Placement

There is limited literature on USGI for medial epicondylosis. Given the proximity of the ulnar nerve to the common flexor tendon there is the potential to accidentally injure the nerve, and case reports have described this complication with LMGI of corticosteroids in this region.[48]

The senior author prefers positioning the patient in a supine position for comfort, although the procedure can be done with the patient seated. The elbow should be flexed and abducted approximately 90°, forearm supine, and the medial aspect of the elbow facing the clinician. The US transducer should be positioned in long axis to the common flexor tendon origin, the needle oriented in plane to the transducer, and the needle advanced in a distal to proximal direction (**Fig. 2**). Similar to injection of the common extensor tendon, the length of the needle is typically 25 to 38 mm, needle may vary from 18 to 25 gauge depending on the indication and goals of the procedure, and injectate volume is typically 2 to 3 mL.

Ulnar Collateral Ligament Disorders

The UCL is the most commonly injured soft tissue structure in overhead throwing athletes, and in one study, accounted for 97% of elbow complaints among baseball pitchers.[49] Surgical management is typically reserved for complete tears of the ligament or partial tears that fail conservative management. However, there is limited literature on nonsurgical management of UCL insufficiency, and only 1 published report to date describes using USGI to treat partial UCL tears. In 2013, Podesta and colleagues[50] presented a series of 34 overhand-throwing athletes with a partial UCL tear confirmed by MRI and treated with a single leukocyte-rich PRP injection under US guidance. Subjects were followed for an average of 70 weeks (range, 11–117 weeks), and the average return to play was 12 weeks (range, 10–15 weeks) postprocedure, with a statistically significant improvement in mean Kerlan-Jobe Orthopaedic Clinical Shoulder and Elbow and Disabilities of the Arm, Shoulder, and Hand scores.

ANTERIOR EVALUATION

The distal biceps brachii tendon and brachialis muscle cross the anterior joint recess before inserting on the radial tuberosity and ulna, respectively. On US, the biceps tendon appears hyperechoic and fibrillary as it crosses the joint, but as it dives deep toward its insertion the tendon appears hypoechoic because of anisotropy artifact, which makes it difficult to assess for pathologic changes in echogenicity, but other pathologic findings include a change in the caliber of the tendon or presence

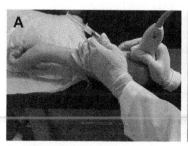 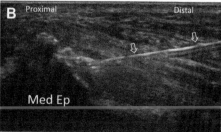

Fig. 2. Technique for US-guided percutaneous injection of the common flexor tendon with a longitudinal, in-plane approach (A). An intratendinous (B) needle placement (*open arrows*) is depicted in the US image, whereas the medial epicondyle (Med Ep) serves as a bony acoustic landmark.

of peritendinous fluid. The anterior evaluation should also include identification of the neurovascular structures before proceeding with an injection.

Distal Biceps Tendinopathy

Distal biceps disorder is uncommon, and a recent retrospective review of a national database estimated the incidence of surgically repaired distal biceps and triceps tendons (which have the same CPT [current procedural terminology] code) at 2.55 cases per 100,000 person-years.[51] Complete distal biceps ruptures require early surgical repair, but the literature on distal biceps tendon partial tears and tendinosis is limited to case series.[52] Peritendinous corticosteroid injections have been advocated for management of partial tears or tendinosis of the distal biceps tendon,[53,54] but carry the potential risk of tendon rupture.[55,56]

The paucity of palpable anatomic landmarks and location of the anterior neurovascular structures makes accurate needle placement challenging. Although various USGI approaches have been described in cadaveric studies,[54] the literature on USGI for distal biceps disorders is otherwise limited to case reports and small cohort studies of intratendinous PRP injections.[57–59]

Sonographic Needle Placement

Because of anisotropy, the distal biceps tendon can be difficult to visualize on US. Sellon and colleagues[54] examined the accuracy of US-guided intratendinous and peritendinous injections of the distal biceps tendon using cadavers and injectable liquid latex. Three intratendinous and 4 peritendinous approaches were studied, using both anterior and posterior windows. The intratendinous injections were successful in 14 of 15 (94%) cases. All 18 peritendinous injections were successful, but 1 anterior approach injection had penetration of the brachial artery. The investigators noted that the posterior approach decreased the risk of vascular injury, but drawbacks included limited proximal peritendinous spread and risk of injectate placement within the supinator muscle. In 1 of the 3 posterior peritendinous approaches, 60% of the injections had latex within the supinator muscle and in close proximity to the posterior interosseous nerve.[54]

The senior author prefers a posterior approach to avoid neurovascular injury. Using the posterior approach, the distal biceps tendon is visualized dorsally between the radius and ulna. The patient is placed in a supine position with the elbow flexed and forearm in full pronation. The transducer is placed in a transverse position between the radius and ulna, and the tendon is visualized as it inserts on the radial tuberosity. Dynamic evaluation of the tendon may be conducted with passive supination and pronation of the forearm. Peritendinous or intratendinous injections are completed using an in-plane approach (**Fig. 3**). The length of the needle is typically 38 to 51 mm, because the target is of intermediate depth, and the needle is typically 18 to 25 gauge depending on the indication and goals of the procedure. Injectate volume is typically 2 to 3 mL.

POSTERIOR EVALUATION

The triceps brachii tendon is composed of a superficial layer (lateral and long heads) and a deep layer (medial head) that blends with the posterior capsule as it inserts on the olecranon process.[42] On US, the normal tendon appears hyperechoic with a characteristic fibrillar pattern. Pathologic changes may include disruption of the tendon fibers (as seen with a partial-thickness or full-thickness tear), or hypoechoic thickening of intact fibers (as seen with tendinosis). Deep to the triceps tendon lies the olecranon

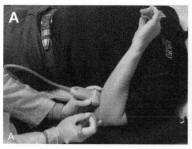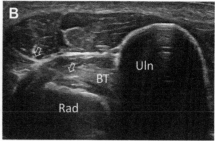

Fig. 3. Technique for US-guided percutaneous injection of the distal biceps tendon with a longitudinal, in-plane approach (*A*). An intratendinous (*B*) needle placement (*open arrows*) is depicted in the US image. BT, biceps tendon; Uln, ulna.

fossa. If clinical suspicion exists, the posterior US evaluation should include assessment of the olecranon bursa superficial to the olecranon process.

Triceps Brachii Disorders

Distal triceps tendon disorder is rare, accounting for less than 1% of all tendon ruptures in the upper limb.[60] Complete tears of the distal triceps tendon are almost uniformly managed surgically[60]; however, the literature is limited on conservative management of partial triceps tendon tears or tendinosis. Similar to the distal biceps tendon, local corticosteroid injections have been associated with subsequent rupture of the triceps tendon.[61,62] One case report has described the successful management of a partial triceps tear with an unguided PRP injection,[63] but otherwise the literature is limited.

Sonographic Needle Placement

The patient is positioned supine, with the elbow flexed to 90° and forearm resting on the abdomen. Alternatively, the patient can be prone with elbow flexed to 90° and forearm hanging off the side of the table. The triceps brachii tendon is located by placing the transducer in long axis on the posterior distal humerus, and peritendinous and intratendinous injections are completed using an in-plane approach. The length of the needle is typically 25 to 38 mm given the superficial nature of the distal triceps brachii tendon; the needle may vary from 18 to 25 gauge depending on the indication and goals of the procedure. Injectate volume is typically 2 to 3 mL.

Elbow Joint Recess

Disorders of the elbow joint can present with a joint effusion. Although the anterior, posterior, or annular recesses can appear distended, the posterior olecranon recess is the most sensitive location to identify pathologic joint fluid with US.[64] US examination should also include an evaluation for synovial hypertrophy and intra-articular loose bodies.

LMGI and aspiration of the elbow joint have been reported in 5 prospective studies (**Table 3**).[6-10] Many of these studies were limited by a small number of subjects and lacked detail regarding the approach. The anterolateral approach was performed in only 1 study, but was the most accurate landmark-guided approach (31 for 31; 100% accuracy).[10] The accuracy of the palpation-guided posterior approach ranged from 64% to 77.5%,[7,9] and 2 studies did not specify the approach used.[6,8]

Table 3
Intra-articular elbow joint injection accuracy

Lead Author (Year)	Injection Approach	US Guidance No (%)	Landmark Guidance No (%)
Balint et al,[6] 2002	Not specified	1 out of 1 (100)	3 out of 8 (37.5)
Jones et al,[8] 1993	Not specified	—	5 out of 6 (83)
Lopes et al,[10] 2008	Anterolateral	—	31 out of 31 (100)
Cunnington et al,[7] 2010	Posterior	10 out of 11 (91)	7 out of 11 (64)
Kim et al,[9] 2013	Posterior	40 out of 40 (100)	31 out of 40 (77.5)
Total	—	51 out of 52 (98.1)	77 out of 96 (80.2)

In all 3 studies that compared the accuracy of USGI with LMGI, the US-guided approach was more accurate. In a 2002 study, Balint and colleagues[6] examined the success of landmark-guided versus US-guided elbow joint aspiration. The approach to the landmark-guided joint aspiration was based on clinical judgment of the treating clinician and not specified by the investigators. The landmark-guided approach was only successful in 3 of 8 (37.5%) cases compared with 1 of 1 US-guided procedure. A 2010 study by Cunnington and colleagues[7] compared the accuracy of LMGI (performed by a senior rheumatologist) with USGI (performed by a trainee) using a posterior approach. The USGI had an accuracy of 91% (10 of 11 cases), compared with 64% (7 of 11 cases) for LMGI. In 2013, Kim and colleagues[9] presented 80 patients with elbow osteoarthritis who underwent USGI or LMGI using a posterior approach, and USGI had an accuracy rate of 100% (40 of 40 cases), whereas the LMGI had a 77.5% accuracy rate (31 of 40 cases).

Sonographic Needle Placement

Intra-articular elbow injections can be performed from a lateral or posterior approach. The lateral approach places the needle tip in the radiocapitellar joint, whereas the posterior approach targets the posterior humeral recess or the space between the olecranon apex and trochlea. Both approaches are discussed here.

Anterolateral Approach

The patient is positioned seated or supine with the elbow flexed to 40°, and the forearm pronated with the palm resting on a table. The transducer is positioned transverse to the radiocapitellar joint (long axis to the radius). The needle should be directed into the radiocapitellar joint using an in-plane approach. The length of the needle is typically 38 to 51 mm given the intermediate depth of the target. A 25-gauge needle is typical for injection only; an 18-gauge is preferred for aspiration. When applicable, injectate volume is typically 2 to 3 mL.

Posterior Approach

The patient is positioned prone with the elbow flexed to 90° and forearm hanging over the edge of the table. The transducer is placed in short axis to the distal triceps tendon over the posterior olecranon fossa. Anechoic fluid in the joint may displace the hyperechoic fat pad posteriorly. The needle can be directed into the joint using an in-plane approach passing beneath the triceps tendon from the lateral to medial side. The ulnar nerve at the medial epicondyle should be visualized before the injection to avoid nerve injury. Needle length, needle gauge, and injectate volume are similar to those used for the anterolateral approach.

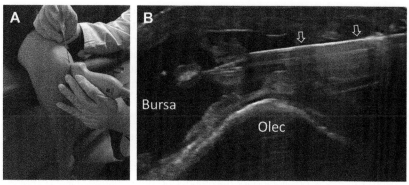

Fig. 4. Technique for US-guided percutaneous aspiration of the olecranon bursa with a longitudinal, in-plane approach (*A*). The US image (*B*) depicts needle placement (*open arrows*) within the olecranon bursa. Olec, olecranon.

Olecranon Bursitis

The olecranon bursa is located superficial to the olecranon process and is generally not sonographically visible in normal states. Common causes of olecranon bursitis include trauma, infection, and inflammatory disorders.[65] There is no standardized approach to management of olecranon bursitis, and nonoperative management of aseptic olecranon bursitis may include observation, nonsteroidal antiinflammatory drugs, compression dressings, and needle aspiration with or without corticosteroid injection. Although septic bursitis requires needle aspiration for diagnosis and appropriate treatment,[66] in cases of aseptic bursitis it is not clear whether the benefits outweigh the risks, including the risk of introducing infection.[67] There is also no clear consensus on the role of corticosteroids for aseptic olecranon bursitis. Although corticosteroid injections are commonly used in clinical practice, a systematic review did not find that corticosteroid injections significantly improved outcome.[65] In addition, case reports have described distal triceps brachii ruptures after unguided corticosteroid injection for olecranon bursitis.[61,62] No studies were found examining the accuracy or clinical outcomes following USGI for olecranon bursitis.

Sonographic Needle Placement

Minimal transducer pressure should be used to avoid displacing any bursal fluid away from the field of view. This minimal pressure can be achieved with a generous layer of gel and floating the transducer over the olecranon. The elbow can be positioned in 90° of flexion, and the transducer placed in a transverse plane to allow better visualization of the bursa. Fluid can be aspirated using an in-plane approach (**Fig. 4**). The length of the needle is typically 25 to 38 mm given the superficial nature of the olecranon bursa. An 18-gauge needle is preferred for completeness of aspiration. When applicable, injectate volume is typically 1 to 3 mL.

SUMMARY

There is a paucity of well-designed studies investigating the accuracy of USGI for elbow disorders. Although several studies have shown improved accuracy when comparing USGI with LMGI of the knee and shoulder, there is a need for more high-level evidence to help guide management in the elbow region. Imaging allows direct visualization of the target and can assist with needle placement. In more advanced procedures, such as percutaneous needle tenotomy or orthobiologic injections, precise needle placement into the pathologic region is important. The lack of US to ensure accurate placement of the injectate limits the conclusions that can be drawn from LMGI studies.[37–39] To properly assess the efficacy of many of these novel treatments for challenging and recalcitrant disorders of the elbow, future studies should use US guidance for confirmation of needle and injectate placement.

REFERENCES

1. Fornalski S, Gupta R, Lee TQ. Anatomy and biomechanics of the elbow joint. Tech Hand Up Extrem Surg 2003;7(4):168–78.
2. Lockard M. Clinical biomechanics of the elbow. J Hand Ther 2006;19(2):72–80.
3. Oxford KL. Elbow positioning for maximum grip performance. J Hand Ther 2000; 13(1):33–6.
4. Alcid JG, Ahmad CS, Lee TQ. Elbow anatomy and structural biomechanics. Clin Sports Med 2004;23(4):503–17, vii.
5. Finnoff JT, Hall MM, Adams E, et al. American Medical Society for Sports Medicine (AMSSM) position statement: interventional musculoskeletal ultrasound in sports medicine. PM R 2015;7(2):151–68.e12.
6. Balint PV, Kane D, Hunter J, et al. Ultrasound guided versus conventional joint and soft tissue fluid aspiration in rheumatology practice: a pilot study. J Rheumatol 2002;29(10):2209–13.
7. Cunnington J, Marshall N, Hide G, et al. A randomized, double-blind, controlled study of ultrasound-guided corticosteroid injection into the joint of patients with inflammatory arthritis. Arthritis Rheum 2010;62(7):1862–9.
8. Jones A, Regan M, Ledingham J, et al. Importance of placement of intra-articular steroid injections. BMJ 1993;307(6915):1329–30.
9. Kim TK, Lee JH, Park KD, et al. Ultrasound versus palpation guidance for intra-articular injections in patients with degenerative osteoarthritis of the elbow. J Clin Ultrasound 2013;41(8):479–85.
10. Lopes RV, Furtado RN, Parmigiani L, et al. Accuracy of intra-articular injections in peripheral joints performed blindly in patients with rheumatoid arthritis. Rheumatology (Oxford) 2008;47(12):1792–4.
11. Connell D, Burke F, Coombes P, et al. Sonographic examination of lateral epicondylitis. AJR Am J Roentgenol 2001;176(3):777–82.
12. Chiavaras MM, Jacobson JA, Carlos R, et al. IMpact of Platelet Rich plasma OVer alternative therapies in patients with lateral Epicondylitis (IMPROVE): protocol for a multicenter randomized controlled study: a multicenter, randomized trial comparing autologous platelet-rich plasma, autologous whole blood, dry needle tendon fenestration, and physical therapy exercises alone on pain and quality of life in patients with lateral epicondylitis. Acad Radiol 2014;21(9):1144–55.
13. Jobe FW, Ciccotti MG. Lateral and medial epicondylitis of the elbow. J Am Acad Orthop Surg 1994;2(1):1–8.
14. Faro F, Wolf JM. Lateral epicondylitis: review and current concepts. J Hand Surg 2007;32A(8):1271–9.
15. Cyriax J, Troisier O. Hydrocortone and soft-tissue lesions. Br Med J 1953;2(4843): 966–8.
16. Krogh TP, Bartels EM, Ellingsen T, et al. Comparative effectiveness of injection therapies in lateral epicondylitis: a systematic review and network meta-analysis of randomized controlled trials. Am J Sports Med 2013;41(6):1435–46.

17. Dogramaci Y, Kalaci A, Savas N, et al. Treatment of lateral epicondilitis using three different local injection modalities: a randomized prospective clinical trial. Arch Orthop Trauma Surg 2009;129(10):1409–14.

18. Lindenhovius A, Henket M, Gilligan BP, et al. Injection of dexamethasone versus placebo for lateral elbow pain: a prospective, double-blind, randomized clinical trial. J Hand Surg Am 2008;33(6):909–19.

19. Newcomer KL, Laskowski ER, Idank DM, et al. Corticosteroid injection in early treatment of lateral epicondylitis. Clin J Sport Med 2001;11(4):214–22.

20. Krogh TP, Fredberg U, Stengaard-Pedersen K, et al. Treatment of lateral epicondylitis with platelet-rich plasma, glucocorticoid, or saline: a randomized, double-blind, placebo-controlled trial. Am J Sports Med 2013;41(3):625–35.

21. Carayannopoulos A, Borg-Stein J, Sokolof J, et al. Prolotherapy versus corticosteroid injections for the treatment of lateral epicondylitis: a randomized controlled trial. PM R 2011;3(8):706–15.

22. Coombes BK, Bisset L, Brooks P, et al. Effect of corticosteroid injection, physiotherapy, or both on clinical outcomes in patients with unilateral lateral epicondylalgia: a randomized controlled trial. JAMA 2013;309(5):461–9.

23. Smidt N, van der Windt DA, Assendelft WJ, et al. Corticosteroid injections, physiotherapy, or a wait-and-see policy for lateral epicondylitis: a randomised controlled trial. Lancet 2002;359(9307):657–62.

24. Verhaar JA, Walenkamp GH, Van Mameren H, et al. Local corticosteroid injection versus Cyriax-type physiotherapy for tennis elbow. J Bone Joint Surg Br 1996; 78(1):128–32.

25. Bisset L, Beller E, Jull G, et al. Mobilisation with movement and exercise, corticosteroid injection, or wait and see for tennis elbow: randomised trial. BMJ 2006; 333(7575):939.

26. McShane JM, Nazarian LN, Harwood MI. Sonographically guided percutaneous needle tenotomy for treatment of common extensor tendinosis in the elbow. J Ultrasound Med 2006;25(10):1281–9.

27. McShane JM, Shah VN, Nazarian LN. Sonographically guided percutaneous needle tenotomy for treatment of common extensor tendinosis in the elbow: is a corticosteroid necessary? J Ultrasound Med 2008;27(8):1137–44.

28. Peerbooms JC, Sluimer J, Bruijn DJ, et al. Positive effect of an autologous platelet concentrate in lateral epicondylitis in a double-blind randomized controlled trial: platelet-rich plasma versus corticosteroid injection with a 1-year follow-up. Am J Sports Med 2010;38(2):255–62.

29. Placzek R, Drescher W, Deuretzbacher G, et al. Treatment of chronic radial epicondylitis with botulinum toxin A. A double-blind, placebo-controlled, randomized multicenter study. J Bone Joint Surg Am 2007;89(2):255–60.

30. Wong SM, Hui AC, Tong PY, et al. Treatment of lateral epicondylitis with botulinum toxin: a randomized, double-blind, placebo-controlled trial. Ann Intern Med 2005; 143(11):793–7.

31. Rabago D, Lee KS, Ryan M, et al. Hypertonic dextrose and morrhuate sodium injections (prolotherapy) for lateral epicondylosis (tennis elbow): results of a single-blind, pilot-level, randomized controlled trial. Am J Phys Med Rehabil 2013;92(7): 587–96.

32. Scarpone M, Rabago DP, Zgierska A, et al. The efficacy of prolotherapy for lateral epicondylosis: a pilot study. Clin J Sport Med 2008;18:248–54.

33. Zeisig E, Ohberg L, Alfredson H. Sclerosing polidocanol injections in chronic painful tennis elbow-promising results in a pilot study. Knee Surg Sports Traumatol Arthrosc 2006;14(11):1218–24.

34. Zeisig E, Fahlström M, Ohberg L, et al. Pain relief after intratendinous injections in patients with tennis elbow: results of a randomised study. Br J Sports Med 2008; 42(4):267–71.

35. Zeisig E, Fahlström M, Ohberg L, et al. A two-year sonographic follow-up after intratendinous injection therapy in patients with tennis elbow. Br J Sports Med 2010;44(8):584–7.

36. Connell DA, Ali KE, Ahmad M, et al. Ultrasound-guided autologous blood injection for tennis elbow. Skeletal Radiol 2006;35(6):371–7.

37. Edwards SG, Calandruccio JH. Autologous blood injections for the refractory lateral epicondylitis. J Hand Surg Am 2003;28(2):272–8.

38. Mishra A, Pavelko T. Treatment of chronic elbow tendinosis with buffered platelet-rich plasma. Am J Sports Med 2006;34(11):1774–8.

39. Mishra AK, Skrepnik NV, Edwards SG, et al. Platelet-rich plasma significantly improves clinical outcomes in patients with chronic tennis elbow a double-blind, prospective, multicenter, controlled trial of 230 patients. Am J Sports Med 2014;42(2):463–71.

40. Connell D, Datir A, Alyas F, et al. Treatment of lateral epicondylitis using skin-derived tenocyte-like cells. Br J Sports Med 2009;43(4):293–8.

41. Stenhouse G, Sookur P, Watson M. Do blood growth factors offer additional benefit in refractory lateral epicondylitis? A prospective, randomized pilot trial of dry needling as a stand-alone procedure versus dry needling and autologous conditioned plasma. Skeletal Radiol 2013;42(11):1515–20.

42. Jacobson JA. Fundamental of musculoskeletal ultrasound. 2nd edition. Philadelphia: Elsevier; 2013.

43. Nazarian LN, McShane JM, Ciccotti MG, et al. Dynamic US of the anterior band of the ulnar collateral ligament of the elbow in asymptomatic major league baseball pitchers. Radiology 2003;227(1):149–54.

44. Leach RE, Miller JK. Lateral and medial epicondylitis of the elbow. Clin Sports Med 1987;6(2):59–72.

45. Lee SS, Kang S, Park NK, et al. Effectiveness of initial extracorporeal shock wave therapy on the newly diagnosed lateral or medial epicondylitis. Ann Rehabil Med 2012;36(5):681–7.

46. Stahl S, Kaufman T. The efficacy of an injection of steroids for medial epicondylitis. J Bone Joint Surg Am 1997;79(11):1648–52.

47. Suresh SP, Ali KE, Jones H, et al. Medial epicondylitis: is ultrasound guided autologous blood injection an effective treatment. Br J Sports Med 2006;40(11):935–9.

48. Stahl S, Kaufman T. Ulnar nerve injury at the elbow after steroid injection for medial epicondylitis. J Hand Surg Br 1997;22(1):69–70.

49. Chen FS, Rokito AS, Jobe FW. Medial elbow problems in the overhead-throwing athlete. J Am Acad Orthop Surg 2001;9(2):99–113.

50. Podesta L, Crow SA, Volkmer D, et al. Treatment of partial ulnar collateral ligament tears in the elbow with platelet-rich plasma. Am J Sports Med 2013;41(7): 1689–94.

51. Kelly MP, Perkinson SG, Ablove RH, et al. Distal biceps tendon ruptures: an epidemiological analysis using a large population database. Am J Sports Med 2015;43(8):2012–7.

52. Hobbs MC, Koch J, Bamberger HB. Distal biceps tendinosis: evidence-based review. J Hand Surg Am 2009;34(6):1124–6.

53. Chew ML, Giuffre BM. Disorders of the distal biceps brachii tendon. Radiographics 2005;25(5):1227–37.

54. Sellon JL, Wempe MK, Smith J. Sonographically guided distal biceps tendon injections: techniques and validation. J Ultrasound Med 2014;33(8):1461–74.
55. Speed CA. Fortnightly review: corticosteroid injections in tendon lesions. BMJ 2001;323(7309):382–6.
56. Vardakas DG, Musgrave DS, Varitimidis SE, et al. Partial rupture of the distal biceps tendon. J Shoulder Elbow Surg 2001;10(4):377–9.
57. Mautner K, Stafford CD 2nd, Nguyen P. Ultrasound-guided distal bicep tendon injection using a posterior approach. PM R 2015;7(9):1007–10.
58. Sanli I, Morgan B, van Tilborg F, et al. Single injection of platelet-rich plasma (PRP) for the treatment of refractory distal biceps tendonitis: long-term results of a prospective multicenter cohort study. Knee Surg Sports Traumatol Arthrosc 2014. [Epub ahead of print].
59. Barker SL, Bell SN, Connell D, et al. Ultrasound-guided platelet-rich plasma injection for distal biceps tendinopathy. Shoulder Elbow 2015;7(2):110–4.
60. Stucken C, Ciccotti MG. Distal biceps and triceps injuries in athletes. Sports Med Arthrosc 2014;22(3):153–63.
61. Mair SD, Isbell WM, Gill TJ, et al. Triceps tendon ruptures in professional football players. Am J Sports Med 2004;32(2):431–4.
62. Stannard JP, Bucknell AL. Rupture of the triceps tendon associated with steroid injections. Am J Sports Med 1993;21(3):482–5.
63. Cheatham SW, Kolber MJ, Salamh PA, et al. Rehabilitation of a partially torn distal triceps tendon after platelet rich plasma injection: a case report. Int J Sports Phys Ther 2013;8(3):290–9.
64. De Maeseneer M, Jacobson JA, Jaovisidha S, et al. Elbow effusions: distribution of joint fluid with flexion and extension and imaging implications. Invest Radiol 1998;33(2):117–25.
65. Sayegh ET, Strauch RJ. Treatment of olecranon bursitis: a systematic review. Arch Orthop Trauma Surg 2014;134(11):1517–36.
66. Raddatz DA, Hoffman GS, Franck WA. Septic bursitis: presentation, treatment and prognosis. J Rheumatol 1987;14(6):1160–3.
67. Weinstein PS, Canoso JJ, Wohlgethan JR. Long-term follow-up of corticosteroid injection for traumatic olecranon bursitis. Ann Rheum Dis 1984;43(1):44–6.
68. AIUM. Practice parameters for the performance of a musculoskeletal ultrasound. American Institute of Ultrasound Medicine; 2012. Available at: http://www.aium.org/resources/guidelines/musculoskeletal.pdf.
69. Wright JG. A practical guide to assigning levels of evidence. J Bone Joint Surg Am 2007;89(5):1128–30.

Ultrasound-Guided Interventional Procedures of the Wrist and Hand

Anatomy, Indications, and Techniques

Sean W. Colio, MD[a], Jay Smith, MD[b,c,d], Adam M. Pourcho, DO[e],*

KEYWORDS

• Ultrasound • Wrist • Hand • Tendinopathy • Arthritis • Ganglion • Finger
• Trigger finger

 Video content accompanies this article at http://www.pmr.theclinics.com.

INTRODUCTION

Tendon-related and joint-related disorders of the wrist and hand region are common clinical conditions that may result in significant functional limitations. When clinically indicated, precisely placed injections can facilitate the diagnosis and management of patients presenting with wrist and hand pain or dysfunction. During the past decade, Ultrasound (US) has emerged as an optimal modality for diagnostic and therapeutic injections about the wrist and hand region because of the superficial location of most wrist and hand targets. More recently, US-guided (USG) interventions have been used for the definitive surgical treatment of selected wrist and hand disorders. This article provides an overview of some of the common indications and techniques for USG procedures of tendon-related and joint-related disorders of the wrist and hand, including:

- Radiocarpal (RC) joint arthritis
- Scaphotrapeziotrapezoidal (STT) joint arthritis

Disclosures: The authors have nothing to disclose.
[a] Department of Physical Medicine and Rehabilitation, Swedish Spine, Sports, and Musculoskeletal Center, Swedish Medical Group, Seattle, WA, USA; [b] Departments of Physical Medicine & Rehabilitation, Mayo Clinic Sports Medicine Center, Mayo Clinic, Rochester, MN, USA; [c] Department Radiology, Mayo Clinic Sports Medicine Center, Mayo Clinic, Rochester, MN, USA; [d] Department Anatomy, Mayo Clinic Sports Medicine Center, Mayo Clinic, Rochester, MN, USA; [e] Department of Physical Medicine and Rehabilitation, Swedish Spine, Sports, and Musculoskeletal Center, Swedish Medical Group, 600 E. Jefferson Street, Suite 300, Seattle, WA 98112, USA
* Corresponding author.
E-mail address: adam.pourcho@swedish.org

Phys Med Rehabil Clin N Am 27 (2016) 589–605
http://dx.doi.org/10.1016/j.pmr.2016.04.003
1047-9651/16/$ – see front matter © 2016 Elsevier Inc. All rights reserved.

- Trapeziometacarpal (TM) (first carpometacarpal [CMC]) joint arthritis
- Metacarpophalangeal (MCP) joint, proximal interphalangeal (PIP) joint, and distal interphalangeal (DIP) joint arthritis
- First dorsal compartment (DC) tenosynovitis (de Quervain syndrome)
- Ganglion cysts
- Stenosing tenosynovitis (trigger finger)

KEY POINTS FOR WRIST AND HAND ULTRASOUND-GUIDED PROCEDURES

- The authors recommend the use of sterile technique with sterile probe covers and sterile gel, but multiple methods have been described to prevent infection during USG interventions.[1]
- For the superficial structures in the wrist and hand, the authors recommend a high-frequency (>10 MHz) linear-array transducer. A small-footprint (hockey stick) transducer may be advantageous, but is not required.
- Although most procedures can be performed sitting or supine, the authors prefer supine positioning for patient comfort and ergonomics, as well as to reduce the risk of vasovagal episodes. Use of an arm board can further optimize positioning during USG procedures.
- Needle selection depends on procedure-specific and patient-specific factors, as well as operator preference. In general, using the smallest-gauge needle to accomplish the procedure minimizes patient discomfort.
- The type and amount of injectate are based on clinical indication, patient-specific factors, and clinician preference. Particulate corticosteroids are hyperechoic with US visualization, and thus may obscure the target when injected. Furthermore, larger particulate steroids may clog smaller-gauge needles.

RADIOCARPAL JOINT

The RC joint is a synovial joint consisting of the articulation between the distal radius and the proximal carpal bones, and is supported by several ligaments and muscle-tendon units, as well as the triangular fibrocartilage complex.[2] A variety of injuries may occur in the wrist, including dislocations, chronic instability, inflammatory arthritis, and osteoarthritis.[3–5] For example, prior scaphoid fractures or scapholunate or lunotriquetral ligament injuries have been shown to predispose to STT joint arthritis.[5,6]

The RC joint is best visualized using a high-frequency linear-array transducer placed dorsally over the distal radius in the anatomic sagittal plane with the wrist pronated and in slight flexion (**Fig. 1**). Common pathologic findings on US include joint effusions, thickening of the synovium/synovitis, articular space narrowing, cortical irregularities, and osteophyte formation.[7]

In patients who fail conservative management for the conditions discussed earlier, diagnostic and/or therapeutic injection of the RC joint may be considered. Furthermore, aspiration of effusion may be indicated as part of the diagnostic work-up for crystalline and inflammatory arthropathies.[3] The reported accuracy rates of palpation-guided (PG) and USG injections into the wrist joint in the clinical setting range from 25% to 97% and 79% to 94% respectively.[8–11]

TECHNIQUE FOR ULTRASOUND-GUIDED RADIOCARPAL JOINT INJECTION

For injection of the RC joint, the patient is placed supine with the hand fully pronated and the wrist in slight flexion with the use of a towel (see **Fig. 1**A). Placing the wrist in

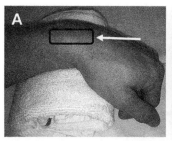
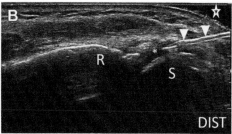

Fig. 1. US-guided RC joint injection. (A) With the forearm pronated and placed over a rolled towel to facilitate wrist flexion, the transducer (*black rectangle*) is placed over the RC joint at the RS joint. The needle trajectory (*solid arrow*) shows an in-plane, distal-to-proximal approach between the second and third DC tendons. (B) Correlative US image showing the hyperechoic needle (*arrowheads*) within the dorsal RS joint (*asterisk*). Notice the use of a gel standoff (*star*) to optimize ergonomics and needle visualization (see also Video 1). DIST, distal; R, radius; S, scaphoid.

flexion opens the dorsal joint recess.[11] The radioscaphoid (RS) joint is the preferred target when injecting the RC joint secondary to its ease of access and lack of significant overlying neurovascular structures.[11] To localize the RS joint, a high-frequency linear-array transducer is placed in the anatomic axial plane over the dorsal wrist at the radial styloid. The transducer is then translated to place Lister's tubercle in the center of the transducer. Following this, the RS joint is visualized by rotating the transducer 90° into the anatomic sagittal plane to produce a long-axis (LAX) view of the joint. The transducer may be slightly rotated to ensure that the needle trajectory is between the second and third extensor compartments, which are separated by Lister's tubercle. This transducer orientation may result in the overlying tendons being oblique to the transducer. Although this results in cortical margins that are less conspicuous, the transducer position is optimized for the injection (see **Fig. 1**). Following localization, a 25-gauge 38-mm needle is inserted via an in-plane distal-to-proximal trajectory toward the articulation, using the distal radius as a bony backstop for the injection. The hypoechoic scaphoid cartilage may or may not be well visualized secondary to transducer orientation (see **Fig. 1**B, Video 1). With this technique, aspiration of an effusion in the wrist joint recess is also possible using a larger-gauge needle. Although not formally described in this article, the joint may alternatively be injected with the transducer in the same position as described earlier using an out-of-plane ulnar-to-radial or radial-to-ulnar trajectory.

SCAPHOTRAPEZIOTRAPEZOIDAL JOINT

The STT joint is a dome-shaped articulation on the radial side of the wrist.[12] The scaphoid is the most radial bone on the proximal carpal row and articulates with the distal radius, capitate, lunate, trapezium, and trapezoid.[13] STT joint arthritis is the second most common pattern of wrist arthritis, observed in up to 15% of radiographic studies and 83.3% of cadaveric specimens.[12,14–20]

The STT joint is best visualized sonographically using a high-frequency linear-array transducer placed over the palmar aspect of the wrist with the forearm supinated. The transducer is first placed parallel (LAX) to the first metacarpal, and then translated proximally until the TM joint and more proximal STT joint are visualized (**Fig. 2**). Common pathologic US findings include joint effusions, synovitis/pannus, articular space narrowing, cortical irregularities, and osteophyte formation.[7,21] The flexor carpi radialis

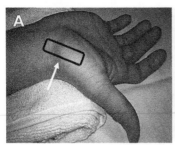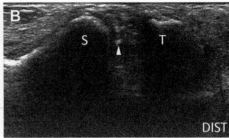

Fig. 2. US-guided STT joint injection. (*A*) With the forearm supinated and placed over a rolled towel to facilitate wrist-thumb extension, the transducer (*black rectangle*) is placed short axis (SAX) to the STT joint. The needle trajectory (*solid arrow*) is via an out-of-plane, radial-to-ulnar approach using a walk-down technique. Care should be taken to remain dorsoradial to the thenar muscles because passing through them can increase patient discomfort. (*B*) Correlative US image showing an out-of-plane view of the hyperechoic needle (*arrowhead*) within the STT joint (see also Video 2). T, trapezium.

(FCR) tendon lies anatomically just palmar and ulnar to the STT joint, and STT joint arthritis may result in FCR tendinopathies and/or tenosynovitis.[22–24] Furthermore, there is often concomitant radiographic and possibly symptomatic TM joint arthritis. Consequently, it is prudent to consider associated pathologic conditions when performing interventional procedures about the STT joint.

In patients who have failed conservative management, such as rest, splitting, activity modification, and medications, injection of the STT joint for diagnostic or therapeutic purposes may be indicated. Smith and colleagues[18] reported sonographically guided and PG injection accuracy rates of 100% and 80% respectively for the STT joint in a cadaveric model.

TECHNIQUE FOR ULTRASOUND-GUIDED SCAPHOTRAPEZIOTRAPEZOIDAL JOINT INJECTION

STT joint injections are accomplished via a palmar out-of-plane approach, with the patient's wrist supinated and the transducer placed LAX over the first metacarpal (see **Fig. 2**A). The STT joint is located by the method described previously, placing the joint in the center of the transducer. Care should be taken to identify the superficial radial artery, which courses adjacent to the palmar surface of the STT.[7,22–24] Following this, a 25-gauge or 27-gauge 38-mm needle is inserted via an out-of-plane radial-to-ulnar approach using a walk-down technique (see **Fig. 2**B, Video 2). The small size of the joint space (usually 1 mL or less), necessitates consideration of injection goals before the procedure. Care must be taken to avoid injecting too much anesthetic into the joint space during the procedure, which may result in insufficient therapeutic injectate in the joint, or overdistention of the joint capsule, which may cause patient discomfort. Alternatively, this injection can be performed via an in-plane radial-to-ulnar approach, with the transducer in the anatomic axial plane.

TRAPEZIOMETACARPAL (FIRST CARPOMETACARPAL) JOINT

The TM joint, also known as the first CMC joint, is the articulation between the first metacarpal and the trapezium, and is crucial for normal thumb mobility.[25] There are several key surrounding structures that need to be taken into consideration when performing TM joint procedures. The superficial radial nerve is located on the radial side of the wrist, and has terminal branches coursing along either side of the TM joint.[26] The radial artery branches into superficial and deep palmar arteries at the anatomic snuffbox just proximal to the TM joint, and its location should be noted before any interventional procedures.[25,27]

The TM joint is the second most common site affected by idiopathic arthritis in the hand, often resulting in a box deformity as well as pain with grasping and fine manipulation.[26] There can be a normal step-off representing radial protrusion of the metacarpal base, which is often accentuated in the setting of arthritis.[18,26] Patients with arthritic changes may also have associated ligamentous laxity.

The TM joint is best visualized using a high-frequency linear-array transducer or small-footprint hockey-stick transducer placed radially over the first metacarpal in the anatomic coronal plane. The transducer is translated proximally until the TM joint is visualized. When static imaging is suboptimal, passive thumb motion reveals the joint margins. Common US findings of TM joint disorder include joint effusion, synovitis/pannus, articular space narrowing, cortical irregularities, radial subluxation, and osteophyte formation.[7,21] For patients with pain that is refractory to conservative management, such as thumb spica, rest, nonsteroidal antiinflammatory drugs (NSAIDs), and occupational therapy, diagnostic or therapeutic injection may be considered. PG injections of the TM joint have been reported to be accurate in 0% to 97% of patients, whereas USG and fluoroscopically guided injections have reported accuracy rates of 94% to 100%.[8,9,28–31]

TECHNIQUE FOR ULTRASOUND-GUIDED TRAPEZIOMETACARPAL (FIRST CARPOMETACARPAL) JOINT INJECTION

The patient is positioned with the forearm in the neutral position (**Fig. 3**A). The injection is performed by first locating the TM joint via the method described earlier and placing the center of the TM joint in the middle of the transducer. A 25-gauge to 27-gauge 32-mm needle is then advanced into the joint using an out-of-plane dorsal-to-palmar approach and a walk-down technique (see **Fig. 3**, Video 3). Occasionally, anatomic

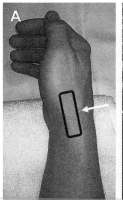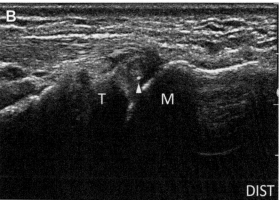

Fig. 3. US-guided TM (first carpometacarpal) joint injection. (A) With the forearm in neutral position, the transducer (*black rectangle*) is placed LAX to the first metacarpal and translated proximally over the TM joint. The needle trajectory (*solid arrow*) is via an out-of-plane, dorsal-to-palmar approach using a walk-down technique. (B) Correlative US image showing an out-of-plane view of the needle tip (*arrowhead*) within the TM (first CMC) joint (see also Video 3). M, first metacarpal.

and pathologic variability may necessitate an out-of-plane palmar-to-dorsal approach or even an in-plane proximal-to-distal or distal-to-proximal approach using a gel standoff. Be aware that using a palmar-to-dorsal approach can result in increased patient discomfort caused by the increased sensitivity of the thenar eminence. Care should be taken to avoid the aforementioned neurovascular structures located within the vicinity of the joint. In addition, clinicians should avoid injecting excessive anesthetic into the joint space during the procedure, which may result in insufficient therapeutic injectate in the joint or overdistention of the joint capsule. In cases of severe osteoarthritis, manipulation of the thumb into a more adducted position may help facilitate a successful injection.

METACARPOPHALANGEAL, INTERPHALANGEAL, PROXIMAL INTERPHALANGEAL, AND DISTAL INTERPHALANGEAL JOINTS

The MCP joints represent the attachments between the metacarpal bones and the proximal phalanges. The proximal interphalangeal (PIP) and DIP joints are the two most distal joints of the hand. The PIP joint connects the proximal and middle phalanx, whereas the DIP joint connects middle and distal phalanx. The thumb is composed of only an interphalangeal (IP) joint and has no middle phalanx. The MCP and IP (PIP, DIP, and thumb IP) joints are stabilized by the collateral ligaments and the flexor-extensor tendons, which are bordered ulnarly and radially by the digital neurovascular bundles.[32]

The MCP and IP joints are the most common joints to be affected by disorders in the hand.[33] Dislocations, sprains, fractures, primary and posttraumatic osteoarthritis, and inflammatory arthropathies are common.[33] These conditions result in pain and dysfunction affecting activities of daily living and occupation in many individuals.

The MCP and IP joints are best viewed using a high-frequency linear-array transducer or small-footprint hockey-stick transducer. Gel standoffs may be used as necessary to optimize visualization. Common pathologic findings include joint effusion, joint erosions, cortical irregularities, synovial thickening/pannus, synovial cysts, articular space narrowing, periarticular ganglia, and osteophyte formation.[7,21]

In patients who have failed conservative management such as paraffin baths, occupational therapy, relative rest, activity modification, and NSAIDs, therapeutic or diagnostic injection may be indicated. Literature regarding accuracy rates for PG and USG injections of the smaller joints of the hand (MCP, IP, DIP, and PIP joints) has reported accuracy rates of 0% to 97% and 94% to 100% respectively.[8,9,28–31]

TECHNIQUE FOR ULTRASOUND-GUIDED METACARPOPHALANGEAL, INTERPHALANGEAL, PROXIMAL INTERPHALANGEAL, AND DISTAL INTERPHALANGEAL JOINT INJECTIONS

The dorsal recesses typically provide the easiest access to the MCP and IP joints. For the dorsal out-of-plane approach, the patient's forearm is pronated and placed over a rolled towel to facilitate finger flexion (**Fig. 4**A). A high-frequency, ideally small-footprint, linear-array transducer is aligned LAX to the phalanges with the target joint placed in the center of the transducer. A 25-gauge or 27-gauge 25-mm needle is inserted via out-of-plane in either an ulnar-to-radial or radial-to-ulnar direction (depending on accessibility) and advanced into the joint space. The amount of injectate is usually small (1 mL or less), because overdistention of the joint capsule usually results in postprocedural pain. Alternatively, an in-plane proximal-to-distal, radial-to-ulnar, or ulnar-to-radial approach to the joint may be used, depending on preference and anatomy.

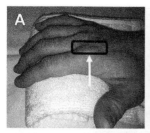
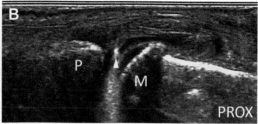

Fig. 4. US-guided MCP joint injection. (A) With the forearm pronated and placed over a rolled towel to facilitate finger flexion, the transducer (*black rectangle*) is placed LAX to the metacarpal and translated distally over the dorsal MCP joint. The needle trajectory in this example (*solid arrow*) is an out-of-plane, radial-to-ulnar approach using a walk-down technique. (B) Correlative US image showing an out-of-plane view of the hyperechoic needle tip (*arrowhead*) within the MCP joint (see also Video 4). M, metacarpal; P, proximal phalanx; PROX, proximal.

FIRST DORSAL COMPARTMENT OF THE WRIST

The first DC of the wrist contains the abductor pollicis longus (APL) and extensor pollicis brevis (EPB) tendons and is anatomically located just radial to the radial styloid. The Lister tubercle at the distal radius separates the second DC (containing the extensor carpi radialis longus and brevis tendons) from the third DC (containing the extensor pollicis longus tendon), is easily palpated, and can serve as a landmark for identifying the first to third DCs. The location of the superficial radial nerve, which travels from palmar to dorsal just proximal to the radial styloid, should be identified before any procedure involving the first DC because it has a variable branching pattern and may be within the planned needle trajectory.[34] The radial artery divides into its superficial and deep branches just deep to the first DC.

First DC stenosing tenosynovitis (de Quervain syndrome) is the most common tendinopathy affecting the wrist and hand.[35,36] The pathophysiology is thought to involve repetitive microtrauma of the first DC, often occupationally or recreationally related, resulting in degenerative and inflammatory changes to the APL and EPB tendons at the level of or just distal to the radial styloid.[37,38] De Quervain syndrome is more common in diabetics and patients with inflammatory arthropathies such as rheumatoid arthritis.[3,9,35] De Quervain syndrome typically presents as pain and tenderness over the radial styloid, with pain exacerbated by wrist and thumb movements, particularly ulnar deviation.[35,37] On physical examination, symptoms can be reproduced with the Finkelstein test (ulnar deviation with the thumb adducted).[39]

The first DC, similar to other superficial structures of the hand, is best viewed using a high-frequency linear-array transducer. The first DC can be identified by placing the wrist in a neutral position and first placing the transducer over the Lister tubercle in the anatomic axial plane to identify the second DC. The transducer is then translated radially along the continuous cortical margin of the radius to identify the first DC tendons lying on the radial aspect of the distal radius. From here, the APL and EPB tendons can be traced proximally to their proximal intersection with the second DC tendons in the dorsal forearm (the site of proximal intersection syndrome) or distally to their insertions.

Common sonographic findings of first DC stenosing tenosynovitis include tendon and synovial sheath thickening, distension of the tendon sheath with anechoic fluid surrounding the tendon, and peritendinous hyperemia on low-flow color Doppler (**Fig. 5B**).[6,7,21] Note that tenosynovial fluid may not be seen at the level of the

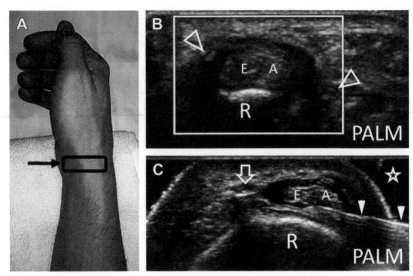

Fig. 5. US-guided first DC injection. (*A*) With the forearm in neutral position, the transducer (*black rectangle*) is placed SAX to the first DC. The needle trajectory in this example (*solid arrow*) is via an in-plane, palmar-to-dorsal approach. (*B*) Correlative US image showing heterogeneic hypoechogenicity of the first DC tendons accompanied by periretinacular hyperemia (*open arrowheads*) at the level of the radial styloid (R). (*C*) US image showing an in-plane view of the hyperechoic needle (*arrowheads*) within the first DC tendon sheath, lying between the tendons (EPB [E] and APL [A]) and radius. Note the use of a gel standoff (*star*) and the close proximity of the dorsally located superficial radial nerve (*open arrow*) (see also Video 5). PALM, palmar.

retinaculum, but more distal because it is likely to flow to regions of less resistance.[7,24] Conservative management includes occupational therapy, workspace/activity modifications, rest, oral and topical NSAIDs, and splinting/bracing.

For patients who fail conservative measures, therapeutic injection may be considered. Stenosing tenosynovitis of the first DC generally responds well to intra–tendon sheath corticosteroid injections, with reported relief in up to 90% of patients.[38,40–42] Recently, platelet-rich plasma and hyaluronic acid injections have also been used with success.[43,44]

Several important anatomic variations warrant consideration with regard to the first DC injection. First DC subcompartmentalization caused by an intracompartment septum may exist in up to 33% of patients, and isolated tenosynovitis of the EPB or, less commonly, the APL can occur.[36,45] Subcompartmentalization has been associated with incomplete response to PG injection because of a lack of flow into the affected subcompartment. USG injection techniques have been shown to be accurate and effective in de Quervain syndrome, with the added benefit of being able to target each subcompartment in the context of a septum.[36,40,46–48] Furthermore, operators should be aware that the APL tendon often has multiple slips that should not be mistaken for longitudinal split tearing.[24,45]

TECHNIQUE FOR ULTRASOUND-GUIDED FIRST DORSAL COMPARTMENT INJECTION

For injection of the first DC, the patient is positioned with the forearm in the neutral position. The first DC is identified as described earlier using a high-frequency, ideally small-footprint, linear-array transducer placed short axis (SAX) to the tendons in the anatomic axial plane at the level of the radial styloid (**Fig. 5**A). The presence of sub-compartmentalization as well as the positions of the superficial radial nerve and radial artery should be noted (**Fig. 5**C).[34,36,45] A 25-gauge or 27-gauge 32-mm needle is inserted via an in-plane, palmar-to-dorsal approach deep to the tendons and adjacent to the radial styloid (see **Fig. 5**C, Video 5). If a septum is present, the needle may be directed into each subcompartment individually. Ideally, injectate (~3 mL) should be seen around both of the tendons. Depending on anatomy and operator preference, this injection may also be done via an in-plane, dorsal-to-palmar approach (although branches of the superficial radial nerve may be in closer proximity using this approach). Alternatively, an in-plane distal-to-proximal or proximal-to-distal approach, with the transducer placed LAX to the tendons, may also be performed. However, these approaches may render selective subcompartment injections difficult in the presence of a septum. Although not discussed in this article, the principles of the injections for the other DCs of the wrist are similar, but are less commonly performed in clinical practice. As always, it is important to have a good understanding of the relevant surrounding anatomy before injection.

GANGLIA

Ganglia are benign, cystic soft tissue fluid collections commonly encountered in the wrist but also occurring around tendon sheaths and other joints throughout the body. They are fluid-filled, generally noncompressible, often septated structures with an epithelial lining and are thought to arise from mucinous degeneration of peri-articular soft tissues.[6,49,50] Of all wrist and hand ganglia, 60% to 70% occur in the dorsal wrist, whereas 15% to 20% occur in the palm.[49,50] The most commonly encountered ganglion in the wrist and hand is associated with the dorsal scapholunate ligament and joint, and may impinge on the posterior interosseous nerve in the fourth DC.[6,50] In the palmar wrist, ganglia are commonly seen overlying the STT joint between the FCR tendon and radial artery, and may impinge on the median nerve.[49,50] Ganglia may also arise from tendons or tendon sheaths.[49] On US, a ganglion appears as a well-defined, anechoic or heterogenous mixed echogenicity, fluid-filled mass often associated with an adjacent joint or ligament via a communicating stalk.[6,7,21,50] Chronic ganglia are more often septated and therefore require precise needle repositioning for complete decompression. It is important to rule out vascular abnormalities with the use of color Doppler before attempting any procedure.

Although many ganglia are asymptomatic, symptoms may occur secondary to compression on neighboring structures. Symptomatic ganglia can be effectively treated with USG aspiration with or without injection.

TECHNIQUE FOR ULTRASOUND-GUIDED GANGLIA INJECTION/ASPIRATION

Given the variability of location of ganglion cysts, patient position depends on the location of the cyst. The wrist and forearm are positioned for patient and operator comfort and to facilitate safe needle advancement for aspiration/injection. A high-frequency linear-array transducer or small-footprint hockey-stick transducer is aligned over the ganglion. A gel standoff may be needed to optimize visualization, and color or power Doppler should be used to identify vascular structures at risk. As with all procedures, a thorough knowledge of the regional anatomy, particularly local neurovascular structures, is necessary to perform a safe and successful procedure. Typically, a large-gauge needle (eg, 18 gauge) is used to penetrate the cyst following delivery of local anesthesia with a smaller-gauge needle (eg, 25 or 27 gauge). Care must be taken to avoid injecting too much anesthetic into the joint space during the procedure, which may result in insufficient therapeutic injectate into the joint, or over-distention of the joint capsule causing postprocedural pain. Because of the high viscosity of ganglion fluid, the use of a large-gauge needle is necessary to facilitate aspiration. In particularly difficult cases, aspiration may be facilitated by lavaging the cyst with local anesthetic or other sterile fluid to reduce the effective viscosity of the ganglion contents. In particularly challenging cases in which fluid cannot be aspirated, fenestration of the cyst walls promotes self-decompression.[50] The needle can also be directed to fenestrate a communicative stalk in an attempt to reduce recurrence. A small amount of corticosteroid can be injected after the procedure to facilitate closure of the cyst and provide symptomatic relief[49] (**Fig. 6**, Video 6).

FLEXOR TENDON SHEATH AT THE FIRST ANNULAR PULLEY

There are 2 tendons responsible for flexion of the fingers: the flexor digitorum superficialis (FDS) and the flexor digitorum profundus. There are 5 annular pulleys (A1–A5), which anatomically are fibro-osseous bands that prevent bowstringing of the flexor tendons during finger flexion.[51] The distal palmar crease can be used for surface localization of the A1 pulley for the ulnar digits and the proximal palmar crease for the radial digits.[51] The A1 pulley is anatomically located palmar to the MCP joint and superficial to the palmar plate.[24,51] The digital neurovascular bundles are located ulnar and radial

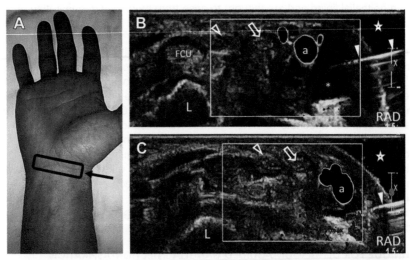

Fig. 6. US-guided ganglion cyst aspiration/injection. (*A*) In this example of a palmar ganglion cyst, the forearm is placed in supination and the transducer (*black rectangle*) is placed in an oblique axial plane with slight counterclockwise rotation. This positioning was necessary to facilitate a safe procedure. The needle trajectory (*solid arrow*) is via an in-plane, radial-to-ulnar approach. (*B*) Correlative US image, with the use of color Doppler, of a palmar ganglion (*asterisk*) arising from the scapholunate joint, showing an in-plane view of the hyperechoic needle (*arrowheads*). Note the ulnar displacement of the median nerve (*open arrowhead*), the FCR tendon (*open arrow*), and the radial artery (a). (*C*) Postaspiration US image shows complete aspiration of the ganglion cyst. The use of a gel standoff (*star*) as well as color Doppler imaging throughout the procedure enhanced its safety, assisting in avoidance of neurovascular structures (see also Video 6). FCU, flexor carpi ulnaris; L, lunate; RAD, radial.

to the flexor tendons, with the digital nerves lying palmar to the vessels when viewed from a palmar perspective.

Although occasionally posttraumatic, stenosing tenosynovitis at the A1 pulley typically develops insidiously and without a definable event.[37,51] Diabetes and inflammatory conditions, such as rheumatoid arthritis and gout, are well-established risk factors.[52,53] Trigger finger typically presents as painful catching of the tendon with or without pain as the finger is flexed and extended. At times the finger can become stuck in flexion and require manual assistance to return to extension. There is frequently a palpable nodule on physical examination, representing a thickened flexor tendon.[37,51]

The A1 pulley is best visualized using a high-frequency linear-array transducer or small-footprint hockey-stick transducer initially placed midpalm in the axial plane over the metacarpal of interest. The transducer is then translated distally while visualizing the associated flexor tendons until a hypoechoic or anechoic ring or belt is encountered surrounding the flexor tendons (**Fig. 7**A, B). This finding occurs approximately between the proximal and distal palmar creases and represents the A1 pulley in its LAX, which is SAX to the flexor tendons. The location of the pulley can be confirmed by rotating 90° to be LAX on the tendons and SAX to the pulley (**Fig. 7**C).[54–58] In this orientation, the pulley can be visualized dynamically during finger flexion in order to document dyskinetic flexor tendon motion or overt triggering at the level of the A1 pulley. The normal A1 pulley is approximately 1 cm in length and has a mean thickness of 0.5 mm.[54–56,58,59] US findings consistent with stenosing tenosynovitis include thickening of the A1 pulley (sometimes associated with neovascularization), tendon enlargement/nodularity, tenosynovitis with or without hyperemia on

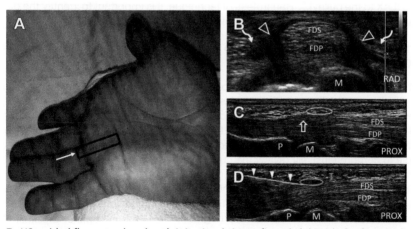

Fig. 7. US-guided flexor tendon sheath injection (trigger finger). (*A*) With the forearm in supination and placed over a rolled towel to facilitate MCP extension, the transducer (*black rectangle*) is placed LAX to the metacarpal and SAX to the MCP joint. The needle trajectory in this example (*solid arrow*) is via an in-plane, distal-to-proximal approach. (*B*) Correlative US image with transducer rotated 90° relative to (*A*), showing a SAX view of the flexor tendons and LAX view of the A1 pulley (*open arrowheads*). The digital neurovascular bundles should be identified (*curved arrows*). (*C*) US image with the same transducer position as (*A*) with the A1 pulley (*oval*) just proximal to the MCP joint. Note the thickening of the FDS tendon (*open arrow*) just distal to the A1 pulley. (*D*) US image showing an in-plane view of the hyperechoic needle (*arrowheads*) within the flexor tendon sheath just deep to the distal A1 pulley (*oval*) (see also Video 7).

color or power Doppler imaging, and abnormal tendon motion during dynamic flexion and extension of the finger with or without triggering.[51,60–62]

Corticosteroid injections have been shown to be beneficial and effective in the treatment of stenosing tenosynovitis at the A1 pulley.[63–66] USG intrasheath injections are more accurate than PG injections and are effective in reducing symptoms at 3-year follow-up.[63,64,67] Intrasheath hyaluronic acid injections have also been shown to reduce triggering at 3-month follow-up.[68] The use of US guidance to perform percutaneous release of the A1 pulley using needles or specialized cutting devices has recently been described with good reults.[65,69–74]

TECHNIQUE FOR ULTRASOUND-GUIDED STENOSING A1 PULLEY INJECTION

The patient is supine on the examination table with the forearm supinated. The wrist and hand are placed in slight dorsiflexion using a rolled up towel or similar support to promote MCP extension, which improves visualization and access to the A1 pulley (see **Fig. 7**A). Visualization can be further enhanced by using a gel standoff. The A1 pulley is identified using the previously described technique. The neurovascular bundles should be identified ulnar and radial to the pulley and underlying flexor tendons, and represent the primary structures at risk during injection or pulley release (see **Fig. 7**B). A high-frequency linear-array transducer, or preferably a small-footprint hockey-stick transducer, is aligned in LAX over the finger flexor tendons with the palmar MCP joint centered on the screen to help visualize the A1 pulley (see **Fig. 7**A, C). A 27-gauge, 32-mm needle is then advanced via a distal-to-proximal approach, placing the needle deep to the distal aspect of the A1 pulley into the tendon sheath (**Fig. 7**D, Video 7). Alternatively, this injection can be performed via an in-plane ulnar-to-radial or radial-to-ulnar approach with the transducer placed SAX to the tendons (LAX to the pulley).[64] Regardless of technique, it is important to identify the digital neurovascular bundle for avoidance before the procedure.

TECHNIQUE FOR ULTRASOUND-GUIDED PERCUTANEOUS A1 PULLEY RELEASE USING HOOK BLADE

Multiple techniques for USG percutaneous A1 pulley release have been described using needles, specialized cutting blades, and other devices.[64,65,69] To the authors' knowledge, no technique has been shown to be superior to any other. As with any technique, a thorough understanding of the relevant anatomy and the goals of the procedure are necessary for procedural success. Although it is beyond the scope of this article to comprehensively review the currently available techniques, a representative technique for USG A1 pulley release is described (**Fig. 8**A).

The wrist and hand are placed in slight dorsiflexion using a rolled up towel or similar support to promote MCP extension (**Fig. 8**B). The transducer is placed LAX to the flexor tendons and SAX to the pulley (**Fig. 8**B, C). The transducer can be rotated 90° SAX to the flexor tendons and LAX to the A1 pulley to identify the ulnar and radial neurovascular bundles (see **Figs. 7**B and **8**E). Following administration of local anesthesia, a 12° hook knife is advanced via an in-plane distal-to-proximal trajectory along the anesthetized track. The blade is maintained palmar to the flexor tendon sheath and A1 pulley, until it passes the proximal edge of the A1 pulley (**Fig. 8**D). The transducer is then rotated 90° into the anatomic axial plane, SAX to the flexor tendons and LAX to the A1 pulley. The blade is then moved dorsally to engage the flexor tendon sheath in the midline, just proximal to the proximal edge of the A1 pulley. A central location is crucial to avoid the digital neurovascular bundles (see **Fig. 8**E). Once engaged, the blade is slowly pulled from proximal to distal to complete transection of the pulley

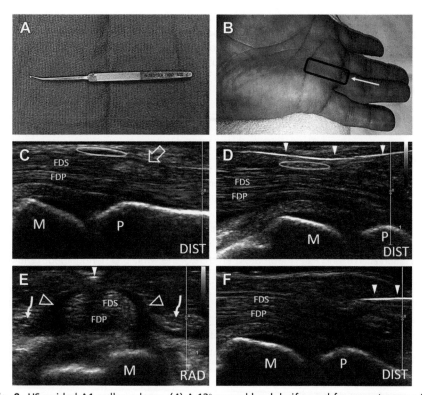

Fig. 8. US-guided A1 pulley release. (*A*) A 12° curved hook knife used for percutaneous A1 pulley release. (*B*) The forearm is supinated and placed over a rolled towel to facilitate MCP extension. The transducer (*black rectangle*) is placed LAX to the flexor tendons and SAX to the MCP joint. The device trajectory in this example (*solid arrow*) is an in-plane, distal-to-proximal approach with an entry point at or near the proximal finger crease. (*C*) Correlative US image showing a LAX view of the flexor tendons and a SAX view of the A1 pulley (*oval*). Note the mixed hyperechoic nodule within the FDS tendon just distal to the pulley (*open arrow*). (*D*) US image with similar orientation to Fig. 8C showing a LAX view of the hyperechoic hook knife (*arrowheads*), superficial to the A1 pulley with its proximal extent proximal to the proximal edge of the A1 pulley. (*E*) US image with transducer rotated 90° relative to (*C* and *D*), showing a SAX view of the flexor tendons. The hyperechoic tip of the hook knife (*arrowheads*) is seen in an out-of-plane view, located centrally with respect to the A1 pulley. The digital neurovascular bundles are shown (*curved arrows*). (*F*) US image with orientation similar to (*C*) and (*D*), showing an in-plane view of the hook knife following A1 pulley release. Compared with (*D*), the device tip (*arrowheads*) is located distal to the A1 pulley, at the proximal phalangeal neck-base junction. Following the procedure, the motion of the tendon can be rechecked dynamically to ensure complete release (see also Video 8).

while continually monitoring the blade position using real-time US guidance using orthogonal imaging SAX and LAX to the flexor tendons (**Fig. 8**F, Video 8). Following successful release, the tendon motion can dynamically be retested to confirm complete release without triggering.

SUMMARY

USG can be used diagnostically or therapeutically on multiple pathologic conditions about the wrist and hand. With their accessibility, increased accuracy, portability, and lack of contraindications, USG injections have several advantages compared with PG injections. As with any procedure, a good understanding of the relevant anatomy helps to facilitate a safe procedure. Therefore, USG should be considered when performing minimally invasive procedures about the wrist and hand.

SUPPLEMENTARY DATA

Supplementary data related to this article can be found online at http://dx.doi.org/10.1016/j.pmr.2016.04.003.

REFERENCES

1. Finnoff J, Hall M, Adams E, et al. American Medical Society for Sports Medicine (AMSSM) position statement: interventional musculoskeletal ultrasound in sports medicine. Br J Sports Med 2015;49(3):145–50.
2. Schmidt HM. Functional anatomy and biomechanics of the wrist joint. Kongressbd Dtsch Ges Chir Kongr 2001;118:399–401 [in German].
3. Rosen A, Weiland AJ. Rheumatoid arthritis of the wrist and hand. Rheum Dis Clin North Am 1998;24(1):101–28.
4. Gaston RG, Loeffler BJ. Sports-specific injuries of the hand and wrist. Clin Sports Med 2015;34(1):1–10.
5. Geissler WB, Burkett JL. Ligamentous sports injuries of the hand and wrist. Sports Med Arthrosc 2014;22(1):39–44.
6. Tagliafico A, Rubino M, Autuori A, et al. Wrist and hand ultrasound. Semin Musculoskelet Radiol 2007;11(2):95–104.
7. Jacobson J. Fundamentals of musculoskeletal ultrasound. 2nd edition. Philadelphia: Saunders; 2013.
8. Balint PV, Kane D, Hunter J, et al. Ultrasound guided versus conventional joint and soft tissue fluid aspiration in rheumatology practice: a pilot study. J Rheumatol 2002;29(10):2209–13.
9. Lopes RV, Furtado RN, Parmigiani L, et al. Accuracy of intra-articular injections in peripheral joints performed blindly in patients with rheumatoid arthritis. Rheumatology (Oxford) 2008;47(12):1792–4.
10. Cunnington J, Marshall N, Hide G, et al. A randomized, double-blind, controlled study of ultrasound-guided corticosteroid injection into the joint of patients with inflammatory arthritis. Arthritis Rheum 2010;62(7):1862–9.
11. Lohman M, Vasenius J, Nieminen O. Ultrasound guidance for puncture and injection in the radiocarpal joint. Acta Radiol 2007;48(7):744–7.
12. White L, Clavijo J, Gilula LA, et al. Classification system for isolated arthritis of the scaphotrapeziotrapezoidal joint. Scand J Plast Reconstr Surg Hand Surg 2010;44(2):112–7.
13. Wolf JM. Treatment of scaphotrapezio-trapezoid arthritis. Hand Clin 2008;24(3):301–6.
14. Crosby EB, Linscheid RL, Dobyns JH. Scaphotrapezial trapezoidal arthrosis. J Hand Surg Am 1978;3(3):223–34.
15. Rogers W, Watson H. Degenerative arthritis at the triscaphe joint. J Hand Surg Am 1990;15(2):232–5.
16. Armstrong AL, Hunter JB, Davis TR. The prevalence of degenerative arthritis of the base of the thumb in post-menopausal women. J Hand Surg Br 1994;19(3):340–1.

17. Moritomo H, Viegas SF, Nakamura K, et al. The scaphotrapezio-trapezoidal joint. Part 1: an anatomic and radiographic study. J Hand Surg Am 2000;25(5): 899–910.
18. Smith J, Brault J, Rizzo M, et al. Accuracy of sonographically guided and palpation guided scaphotrapeziotrapezoid joint injections. J Ultrasound Med 2011; 30(11):1509–15.
19. Kapoutsis DV, Dardas A, Day CS. Carpometacarpal and scaphotrapeziotrapezoid arthritis: arthroscopy, arthroplasty, and arthrodesis. J Hand Surg Am 2011; 36(2):354–66.
20. Bhatia A, Pisoh T, Touam C, et al. Incidence and distribution of scaphotrapezotrapezoidal arthritis in 73 fresh cadaveric wrists. Ann Chir Main Memb Super 1996; 15(4):220–5.
21. Bianchi S. Ultrasound of the musculoskeletal system. 1st edition. Germany: Springer Verlag; 2007.
22. Luong DH, Smith J, Bianchi S. Flexor carpi radialis tendon ultrasound pictorial essay. Skeletal Radiol 2014;43(6):745–60.
23. Smith J, Kakar S. Combined flexor carpi radialis tear and flexor carpi radialis brevis tendinopathy identified by ultrasound: a case report. PM R 2014;6(10):956–9.
24. Chiavaras MM, Jacobson JA, Yablon CM, et al. Pitfalls in wrist and hand ultrasound. AJR Am J Roentgenol 2014;203(3):531–40.
25. Iagnocco A, Coari G. Usefulness of high resolution US in the evaluation of effusion in osteoarthritic first carpometacarpal joint. Scand J Rheumatol 2000; 29(3):170–3.
26. Swigart CR. Arthritis of the base of the thumb. Curr Rev Musculoskelet Med 2008; 1(2):142–6.
27. Hazani R, Engineer NJ, Cooney D, et al. Anatomic landmarks for the first dorsal compartment. Eplasty 2008;8:e53.
28. Pollard M, Cermak M, Buck W, et al. Accuracy of injection into the basal joint of the thumb. Am J Orthop (Belle Mead NJ) 2007;36(2):204–6.
29. Raza K, Lee CY, Pilling D, et al. Ultrasound guidance allows accurate needle placement and aspiration from small joints in patients with early inflammatory arthritis. Rheumatology (Oxford) 2003;42(8):976–9.
30. Umphrey GL, Brault JS, Hurdle MF, et al. Ultrasound-guided intra-articular injection of the trapeziometacarpal joint: description of technique. Arch Phys Med Rehabil 2008;89(1):153–6.
31. Jones A, Regan M, Ledingham J, et al. Importance of placement of intra-articular steroid injections. BMJ 1993;307(6915):1329–30.
32. Moran C. Anatomy of the hand. Phys Ther 1989;69(12):1007–13.
33. Leung GJ, Rainsford KD, Kean WF. Osteoarthritis of the hand I: aetiology and pathogenesis, risk factors, investigation and diagnosis. J Pharm Pharmacol 2014;66(3):339–46.
34. Samarakoon LB, Lakmal KC, Thillainathan S, et al. Anatomical relations of the superficial sensory branches of the radial nerve: a cadaveric study with clinical implications. Patient Saf Surg 2011;5(1):28.
35. Rettig AC. Athletic injuries of the wrist and hand: part II: overuse injuries of the wrist and traumatic injuries to the hand. Am J Sports Med 2004;32(1):262–73.
36. Choi SJ, Ahn JH, Lee YJ, et al. de Quervain disease: US identification of anatomic variations in the first extensor compartment with an emphasis on subcompartmentalization. Radiology 2011;260(2):480–6.
37. Vuillemin V, Guerini H, Bard H, et al. Stenosing tenosynovitis. J Ultrasound 2012; 15(1):20–8.

38. Sawaizumi T, Nanno M, Ito H. De Quervain's disease: efficacy of intra-sheath triamcinolone injection. Int Orthop 2007;31(2):265–8.
39. Kutsumi K, Amadio PC, Zhao C, et al. Finkelstein's test: a biomechanical analysis. J Hand Surg Am 2005;30(1):130–5.
40. Jeyapalan K, Choudhary S. Ultrasound-guided injection of triamcinolone and bupivacaine in the management of De Quervain's disease. Skeletal Radiol 2009;38(11):1099–103.
41. Anderson B, Manthey R, Brouns M. Treatment of De Quervain's tenosynovitis with corticosteroids. A prospective study of the response to local injection. Arthritis Rheum 1991;34(7):793–8.
42. Jirarattanaphochai K, Saengnipanthkul S, Vipulakorn K, et al. Treatment of de Quervain disease with triamcinolone injection with or without nimesulide. A randomized, double-blind, placebo-controlled trial. J Bone Joint Surg Am 2004;86-A(12):2700–6.
43. Orlandi D, Corazza A, Fabbro E, et al. Ultrasound-guided percutaneous injection to treat de Quervain's disease using three different techniques: a randomized controlled trial. Eur Radiol 2015;25(5):1512–9.
44. Peck E, Ely E. Successful treatment of de Quervain tenosynovitis with ultrasound-guided percutaneous needle tenotomy and platelet-rich plasma injection: a case presentation. PM R 2013;5(5):438–41.
45. Motoura H, Shiozaki K, Kawasaki K. Anatomical variations in the tendon sheath of the first compartment. Anat Sci Int 2010;85(3):145–51.
46. Hajder E, de Jonge MC, van der Horst CM, et al. The role of ultrasound-guided triamcinolone injection in the treatment of de Quervain's disease: treatment and a diagnostic tool? Chir Main 2013;32(6):403–7.
47. Kume K, Amano K, Yamada S, et al. In de Quervain's with a separate EPB compartment, ultrasound-guided steroid injection is more effective than a clinical injection technique: a prospective open-label study. J Hand Surg Eur Vol 2012;37(6):523–7.
48. McDermott JD, Ilyas AM, Nazarian LN, et al. Ultrasound-guided injections for de Quervain's tenosynovitis. Clin Orthop Relat Res 2012;470(7):1925–31.
49. Gude W, Morelli V. Ganglion cysts of the wrist: pathophysiology, clinical picture, and management. Curr Rev Musculoskelet Med 2008;1(3–4):205–11.
50. Wang G, Jacobson JA, Feng FY, et al. Sonography of wrist ganglion cysts: variable and noncystic appearances. J Ultrasound Med 2007;26(10):1323–8 [quiz: 1330–1].
51. Fiorini HJ, Santos JB, Hirakawa CK, et al. Anatomical study of the A1 pulley: length and location by means of cutaneous landmarks on the palmar surface. J Hand Surg Am 2011;36(3):464–8.
52. Zyluk A, Puchalski P. Hand disorders associated with diabetes: a review. Acta Orthop Belg 2015;81(2):191–6.
53. Park IJ, Lee YM, Kim HM, et al. Multiple etiologies of trigger wrist. J Plast Reconstr Aesthet Surg 2016;69(3):335–40.
54. Guerini H, Pessis E, Theumann N, et al. Sonographic appearance of trigger fingers. J Ultrasound Med 2008;27(10):1407–13.
55. Wilhelmi BJ, Snyder NT, Verbesey JE, et al. Trigger finger release with hand surface landmark ratios: an anatomic and clinical study. Plast Reconstr Surg 2001;108(4):908–15.
56. Boutry N, Titecat M, Demondion X, et al. High-frequency ultrasonographic examination of the finger pulley system. J Ultrasound Med 2005;24(10):1333–9.

57. Serafini G, Derchi LE, Quadri P, et al. High resolution sonography of the flexor tendons in trigger fingers. J Ultrasound Med 1996;15(3):213–9.
58. Martinoli C, Bianchi S, Nebiolo M, et al. Sonographic evaluation of digital annular pulley tears. Skeletal Radiol 2000;29(7):387–91.
59. Serafini G, Sconfienza L, Lacelli F, et al. Rotator cuff calcific tendonitis: short-term and 10-year outcomes after two-needle us-guided percutaneous treatment–nonrandomized controlled trial. Radiology 2009;252(1):157–64.
60. Sato J, Ishii Y, Noguchi H, et al. Sonographic appearance of the flexor tendon, volar plate, and A1 pulley with respect to the severity of trigger finger. J Hand Surg Am 2012;37(10):2012–20.
61. van Tongel A, MacDonald P, Leiter J, et al. A cadaveric study of the structural anatomy of the sternoclavicular joint. Clin Anat 2012;25(7):903–10.
62. Barbaix E, Lapierre M, Van Roy P, et al. The sternoclavicular joint: variants of the discus articularis. Clin Biomech (Bristol, Avon) 2000;15(Suppl 1):S3–7.
63. Chambers RG Jr. Corticosteroid injections for trigger finger. Am Fam Physician 2009;80(5):454.
64. Bodor M, Flossman T. Ultrasound-guided first annular pulley injection for trigger finger. J Ultrasound Med 2009;28(6):737–43.
65. Smith J, Rizzo M, Lai JK. Sonographically guided percutaneous first annular pulley release: cadaveric safety study of needle and knife techniques. J Ultrasound Med 2010;29(11):1531–42.
66. Marks MR, Gunther SF. Efficacy of cortisone injection in treatment of trigger fingers and thumbs. J Hand Surg Am 1989;14(4):722–7.
67. Lee D, Han S, Park J, et al. Sonographically guided tendon sheath injections are more accurate than blind injections: implications for trigger finger treatment. J Ultrasound Med 2011;30(2):197–203.
68. Liu DH, Tsai MW, Lin SH, et al. Ultrasound-guided hyaluronic acid injections for trigger finger: a double-blinded, randomized controlled trial. Arch Phys Med Rehabil 2015;96(12):2120–7.
69. Paulius KL, Maguina P. Ultrasound-assisted percutaneous trigger finger release: is it safe? Hand (N Y) 2009;4(1):35–7.
70. Gulabi D, Cecen GS, Bekler HI, et al. A study of 60 patients with percutaneous trigger finger releases: clinical and ultrasonographic findings. J Hand Surg Eur. 2014, 39: 699–703. J Hand Surg Eur Vol 2015;40(1):103–4.
71. Mishra SR, Gaur AK, Choudhary MM, et al. Percutaneous A1 pulley release by the tip of a 20-g hypodermic needle before open surgical procedure in trigger finger management. Tech Hand Up Extrem Surg 2013;17(2):112–5.
72. Habbu R, Putnam MD, Adams JE. Percutaneous release of the A1 pulley: a cadaver study. J Hand Surg Am 2012;37(11):2273–7.
73. Saengnipanthkul S, Sae-Jung S, Sumananont C. Percutaneous release of the A1 pulley using a modified Kirschner wire: a cadaveric study. J Orthop Surg (Hong Kong) 2014;22(2):232–5.
74. Wang H, Zeng H, Wu H, et al. Percutaneous release of trigger finger with L shaped hollow needle knife. Zhongguo Xiu Fu Chong Jian Wai Ke Za Zhi 2012;26(1):14–6.

Ultrasound-Guided Hip Procedures

Jeffrey M. Payne, MD*

KEYWORDS

- Ultrasound • Injection • Hip joint • Iliopsoas bursa • Trochanteric bursa
- Ischial bursa • Piriformis muscle

KEY POINTS

- The differential diagnosis for hip pain is extensive and includes intra-articular and extra-articular pathologic conditions, and referred pain from the lumbar spine and pelvis.
- Ultrasound (US) is commonly used to evaluate hip region pathologic conditions and to guide interventions in the hip region for diagnostic and therapeutic purposes.
- US confers many advantages compared with other commonly used imaging modalities, including real-time visualization of muscles, tendons, bursae, neurovascular structures, and the needle during an intervention.
- US-guided injection techniques have been described for many commonly performed procedures in the hip region, and many studies have been performed demonstrating the safety and accuracy of these techniques.

 Video content accompanies this article at http://www.pmr.theclinics.com.

INTRODUCTION

The differential diagnosis for hip pain is extensive and includes intra-articular and extra-articular pathologic conditions, and referred pain from the lumbar spine and pelvis.[1] Ultrasound (US) is commonly used to evaluate pathologic conditions and to guide interventions in the hip region for diagnostic and therapeutic purposes.[2–15] Indications for performing interventions with image guidance include the proximity of neurovascular structures, lack of palpable anatomic landmarks, large body habitus, deep location of target, and the heightened need for accuracy when performing a diagnostic injection. In comparison with computed tomography (CT) and fluoroscopy, US does not produce ionizing radiation, has no absolute contraindications, does not require contrast agents, and is able to be performed with less expensive and more portable

Disclosures: The author has no commercial or financial conflicts of interest.
Physical Medicine and Rehabilitation, Mayo Clinic Health System, 300 State Avenue, Faribault, MN 55021, USA
* 200 First Street SW, Rochester, Minnesota 55905, USA
E-mail address: payne.jeffrey@mayo.edu

Phys Med Rehabil Clin N Am 27 (2016) 607–629
http://dx.doi.org/10.1016/j.pmr.2016.04.004
1047-9651/16/$ – see front matter © 2016 Elsevier Inc. All rights reserved.

equipment.[9] US can identify bony acoustic landmarks and provides high-resolution soft tissue imaging, allowing for real-time visualization of muscles, tendons, and fascial planes.[7,8] US also allows for visualization of important neurovascular structures to assist in the prevention of injection-related complications.[7,8] This article describes the techniques for performing US-guided procedures in the hip region, including intra-articular hip injection, iliopsoas bursa injection, greater trochanter bursa injection, ischial bursa injection, and piriformis muscle injection. In addition, the common indications, pitfalls, accuracy, and efficacy of these procedures are addressed.

ULTRASOUND-GUIDED HIP JOINT INJECTION
Diagnostic Criteria

Intra-articular causes of hip pain include osteoarthritis, acetabular labral tears, femoroacetabular impingement, loose bodies, and ligamentum teres tears.[1] Hip osteoarthritis is most often symptomatic with weight-bearing activities but may also cause pain at night. Management options include activity modification, weight loss, analgesics, physical therapy, intra-articular steroids, viscosupplementation, and total hip arthroplasty.[16]

Patients with intra-articular pathologic conditions may not have signs and symptoms clearly localized to the hip joint. Often, patients will have concomitant knee or spine conditions, making a definite diagnosis difficult. In these patients, an intra-articular injection of local anesthetic can be useful in confirming hip pathologic conditions and has been associated with predicting a good surgical outcome.[14,15] Hip joint corticosteroid injections have been shown to decrease pain, stiffness, and disability in patients with hip osteoarthritis.[17] Intra-articular hip injections with hyaluronic acid products have also been performed in patients with hip osteoarthritis.[18,19]

Intra-articular hip injections have been performed with palpation guidance using anatomic landmarks, as well as with image guidance using fluoroscopy, CT, and US.[20–28] Hip joint injections are technically challenging to perform because of the deep location of the joint, variable body habitus, and the adjacent femoral neurovascular bundle. Therefore, image guidance has been recommended to ensure safety and accurate needle placement.[20] Sonography can identify the femoral neurovascular bundle, reveal intra-articular fluid collections, and visualize needle passage into the hip joint.[26] Byrd and colleagues[23] reported that patients found in-office US-guided hip injections more convenient and less painful than the same procedure under fluoroscopy. US-guided hip joint injections have been shown to have an excellent safety profile. Sofka and colleagues[28] reported no major complications with 358 US-guided hip joint aspirations or injections, including no inadvertent vascular or femoral nerve puncture. Also, Migliore and colleagues[19] performed 4002 intra-articular hip injections with hyaluronan products and reported no major complications.

Several studies have been performed confirming the accuracy of US-guided hip joint injections.[10,18,26,29] A recent meta-analysis revealed that US-guided hip joint injections are significantly more accurate than landmark-guided intra-articular hip injections.[30] In addition, a systematic literature review for a position statement by the American Medical Society for Sports Medicine found four level 1 studies of US-guided hip injections with a mean accuracy of 99%.[31] Two level 2 studies were identified for landmark-guided hip injections with a mean accuracy of 73%.[31]

Several studies have evaluated the efficacy of US-guided hip joint injections.[18,27,32,33] Micu and colleagues[27] found that US-guided hip intra-articular corticosteroid injections are efficacious in achieving pain control in patients with hip osteoarthritis. Furtado and colleagues[33] compared the short-term effectiveness of

US-guided versus fluoroscopy-guided intra-articular hip injections in patients with synovitis caused by autoimmune or degenerative disorders. For almost all variables that they evaluated, including pain, they found no statistically significant difference between the fluoroscopy-guided and US-guided hip injection groups.[33]

Injection Technique

In preparation for performing a US-guided hip joint injection, the patient is placed in the supine position with the hip in neutral rotation.[6] Preprocedure US evaluation of the anterior hip is usually performed with a low-frequency curvilinear-array transducer. The transducer is placed anteriorly in the oblique sagittal plane, parallel to the femoral neck. This allows visualization of the femoral head-neck junction as well as the overlying hyperechoic iliofemoral ligament and joint capsule.[6] This image is also optimal to evaluate for an effusion in the anterior joint recess.[13] The anterior capsule extends inferiorly from the acetabulum and labrum to inserts on the intertrochanteric line, although some fibers are reflected superiorly along the femoral neck to attach at the femoral head-neck junction.[34] Both the anterior and posterior layers measure between 2 to 3 mm in thickness. A normal amount of fluid between the layers should be less than 2 mm and, in the absence of a hip joint effusion, the 2 layers of the capsule are visualized together as a hyperechoic line.[5] A thin layer of hypoechoic hyaline articular cartilage is visualized covering the hyperechoic surface of the femoral head.[5] The anterior acetabular labrum is visualized as a hyperechoic, compact, triangular structure.[35] After identification of the hip joint, the transducer is then rotated into the transverse plane and moved medially to identify the femoral neurovascular bundle.[6] Special consideration should also be taken to also identify the ascending branch of the lateral femoral circumflex artery because this may be in the path of the planned trajectory of the needle (**Fig. 1**). After confirming the position of the neurovascular structures, the transducer is again placed in the oblique-sagittal plane to optimize visualization of the femoral head-neck junction (**Fig. 2**). At this point, the skin at the inferior end of the transducer is marked with a marking pen and the area is prepped in the usual sterile manner.[6] Following the delivery of local anesthesia, a 22-gauge 64-mm to 89-mm needle is advanced under direct US visualization into the anterior joint recess at the junction of the femoral head and neck (**Fig. 3**).[6] The needle can be felt to pass through the iliofemoral ligament and enter the hip joint (Video 1).[6] The injectate is then delivered while visualizing the injectate flow with real-time sonographic imaging.

ULTRASOUND-GUIDED ILIOPSOAS BURSA INJECTION
Diagnostic Criteria

The main action of the psoas and iliacus muscles is to flex the thigh.[36] The main iliopsoas tendon inserts on the lesser trochanter, although the lateral fibers of the iliacus travel parallel to the iliopsoas tendon and insert directly onto the proximal femoral shaft without a tendon.[3,37] The iliopsoas musculotendinous unit and iliopsoas bursa are subject to mechanical stress with their close proximity to the acetabular rim and hip joint.[38] This can lead to iliopsoas tendinosis or tear. Iliopsoas tendon pathologic conditions may be accompanied by abnormal tendon movement and the source of internal snapping hip.[39] The tendon may be the cause of anterior hip pain after a total hip arthroplasty secondary to friction with the anterior margin of the acetabular cup or impingement on the collar of the femoral prosthesis.[40] With its location between the deep surface of the iliopsoas tendon and acetabular rim and hip joint, iliopsoas bursopathy may accompany iliopsoas tendon pain.[38] Because of the communication

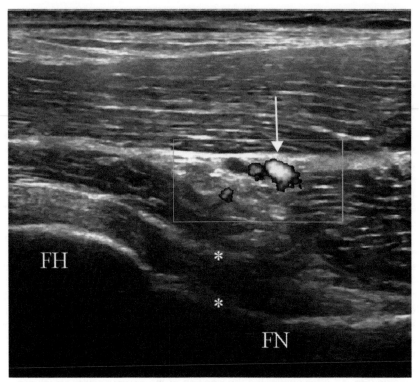

Fig. 1. Anterior oblique sagittal view of the anterior hip joint with lateral femoral circumflex vasculature indicated by the arrow. The asterisks show the anterior joint recess. FH, femoral head; FN, femoral neck. (*Courtesy of* Mayo Foundation for Medical Education and Research, Rochester, MN; with permission.)

between the hip joint and iliopsoas bursa in some individuals, iliopsoas distention is frequently related to hip joint pathologic conditions occurring from various causes, including rheumatoid arthritis, osteoarthritis, villonodular synovitis, synovial chondromatosis, and septic arthritis.[41] Iliopsoas bursitis may also represent a primary pathologic condition, typically related to a previous trauma or overuse syndrome.[41]

Image-guided injections can aid in the diagnosis and treatment of iliopsoas disorders.[38] It is important to be able to perform precise diagnostic iliopsoas injections to identify the source of pain. Iliopsoas injections have been performed with fluoroscopic guidance[42,43] and commonly with US guidance secondary to its excellent soft tissue resolution.[38] US-guided iliopsoas bursa injections have been shown to provide pain relief and predict a good outcome after surgical iliopsoas tendon release for those patients with anterior hip pain and a suspected snapping iliopsoas tendon.[44] Also, US-guided iliopsoas peritendon injections have been described in patients with anterior hip pain following total hip arthroplasty.[40,45,46]

Injection Technique

In preparation for performing a US-guided iliopsoas bursa injection, the patient is placed in the supine position with the hip in neutral rotation. Preprocedure US evaluation of the iliopsoas region is usually performed with a medium-frequency or low-frequency linear-array transducer. The transducer is initially placed in the transverse

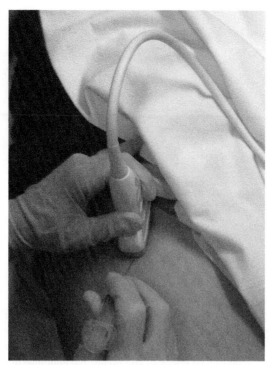

Fig. 2. Anterior oblique sagittal transducer and needle position for an in-plane hip joint injection. (*Courtesy of* Mayo Foundation for Medical Education and Research, Rochester, MN; with permission.)

plane over the femoral head. The transducer is then translated superiorly and angled parallel to the inguinal ligament in the oblique axial plane.[2] At the proximal aspect of the femoral head, the bony contours of the femoral head and acetabulum, along with the iliopsoas muscle and tendon, can be visualized (**Fig. 4**). Toggling the transducer may be necessary to optimize visualization of the iliopsoas tendon secondary to anisotropy. Moving the transducer more superiorly allows visualization of the ilium at the level of the iliopectineal eminence and continued imaging of the iliopsoas muscle and tendon (**Fig. 5**). If a snapping iliopsoas tendon is suspected, a US examination of the iliopsoas tendon can be performed while the patient performs the maneuver that creates the snapping. If a patient cannot reproduce the snapping, a US examination can be performed as the hip is moved from flexion, external rotation, and abduction into full extension, adduction, and internal rotation.[44] Preprocedure scanning includes evaluation for anechoic or hypoechoic distention of the iliopsoas bursa and if present, assessment of a communication between the bursa and the hip joint.

Once preprocedure scanning is complete, the transducer is placed transverse to the iliopsoas tendon in the oblique axial plane, parallel to the inguinal ligament, and superior to the femoral head (**Fig. 6**). The skin at the lateral edge of the transducer is marked with a marking pen and the area is prepped in the usual sterile manner. Following the delivery of local anesthesia, a 22-gauge 89-mm needle is advanced in-plane with the transducer, using a lateral to medial approach.[2] The needle is then advanced under direct US guidance to the deep lateral portion of the iliopsoas tendon where it is directed between the deep surface of the iliopsoas tendon and the superficial surface

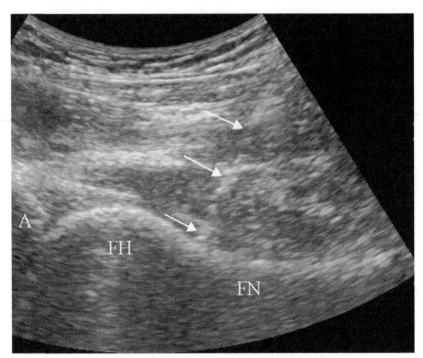

Fig. 3. Anterior oblique sagittal US image of an in-plane hip joint injection. The arrows indicate the needle. A, acetabulum; FH, femoral head; FN, femoral neck. (*Courtesy of* Mayo Foundation for Medical Education and Research, Rochester, MN; with permission.)

of the ilium at the level of the iliopectineal eminence, or alternatively between the iliopsoas tendon and acetabular rim (**Fig. 7**). As the injectate is delivered, fluid will be seen between the iliopsoas tendon and ilium, as well as on the medial side of the iliopsoas tendon (Video 2).[38] Hydrodissection may be useful to identify the plane deep to the iliopsoas tendon but superficial to the hip capsule to avoid inadvertent capsule penetration.[38]

ULTRASOUND-GUIDED GREATER TROCHANTERIC BURSA INJECTION
Diagnostic Criteria

The greater trochanter is a large protuberance that is part of the proximal femur and arises from the junction of the femoral neck and shaft.[47] Four distinct greater trochanter facets have been described: the anterior facet, lateral facet, posterior facet, and superoposterior facet.[48,49] Seven muscles attach to the greater trochanter. The gluteus minimus inserts on the anterior facet, the gluteus medius inserts on both the lateral and superoposterior facets, the piriformis inserts superomedially without a specific facet attachment, the obturator externus inserts medially in the trochanteric fossa, and the obturator internus and superior and inferior gemelli also insert more medially adjacent to the trochanteric fossa.[47–51] Three bursa in the region of the greater trochanter have been described.[47,50,52] The subgluteus minimus bursa is located between the anterior facet and gluteus minimus tendon, the subgluteus medius bursa is located between the lateral facet and gluteus medius tendon, and the subgluteus maximus (greater trochanteric) bursa is located over the posterior and lateral

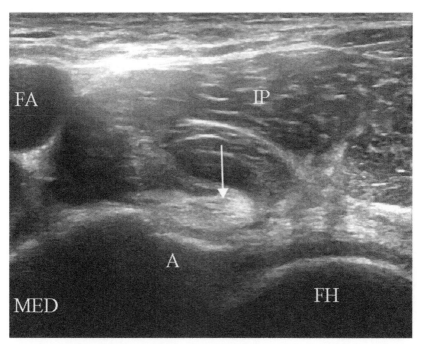

Fig. 4. Transverse oblique US image at the proximal aspect of the femoral head demonstrating the iliopsoas tendon (*arrow*). A, acetabulum; FA, femoral artery; FH, femoral head; IP, iliopsoas muscle; MED, medial. (*Courtesy of* Mayo Foundation for Medical Education and Research, Rochester, MN; with permission.)

facets.[48–50] **Fig. 8** illustrates the 4 greater trochanter facets, the attachment sites of the gluteus medius and minimus tendons, and the location of the regional bursae.[48]

Greater trochanter pain syndrome (GTPS) is a relatively common condition found to affect 17.6% of adults in a large observational study.[53] People with GTPS have high levels of pain, physical impairment, and decreased quality of life.[54] GTPS is a clinical entity that includes several disorders of the lateral hip, including greater trochanteric bursitis, gluteus medius and minimus tendinosis and tears, and snapping hip.[47,50] An anatomic dissection study supported the theory that the greater trochanteric bursa can develop from excessive friction between the greater trochanter and the gluteus maximus.[55] However, histologic analysis of greater trochanteric bursa tissue removed from patients undergoing total hip arthroplasty revealed no signs of acute or chronic inflammation, adding evidence that inflammation or bursitis plays a limited role in GTPS.[56] US and MRI can be used to evaluate the structures of the lateral hip in people with GTPS and most often reveal pathologic conditions involving the gluteus medius and minimus tendons, including tendinosis, calcifications, and tears.[49,50,57] Initial treatment of GTPS involves conservative measures and includes activity modification, ice, weight loss, and physical therapy to address strength and flexibility deficits.[50,52]

Although GTPS is not typically caused by bursitis alone, many patients experience pain relief for a period of several weeks to months following an injection of corticosteroid and local anesthetic into the greater trochanteric bursa.[52] These injections have been performed using a landmark based technique,[52,58] fluoroscopic guidance,[59] and US guidance.[12] McEvoy and colleagues[12] demonstrated that US-guided corticosteroid injections into the greater trochanteric bursa may be more effective than

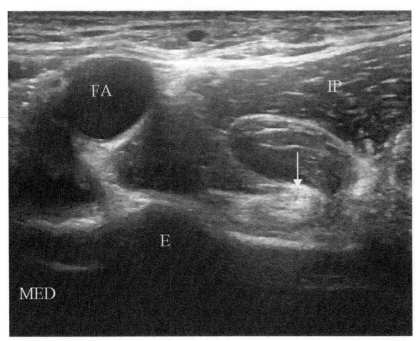

Fig. 5. Transverse oblique US image superior to the femoral head demonstrating the iliopsoas tendon (*arrow*). E, iliopectineal eminence; FA, femoral artery; IP, iliopsoas muscle; MED, medial. (*Courtesy of* Mayo Foundation for Medical Education and Research, Rochester, MN; with permission.)

US-guided corticosteroid injections into the subgluteus medius bursa for treatment of GTPS. Other US-guided treatments that directly target the area of the pathologic condition have been described and may be considered, including percutaneous needle tenotomy, injection of autologous platelet-rich plasma or whole blood, prolotherapy, and others.[50,60,61] Randomized controlled trials comparing the efficacy of these treatment options are needed to better determine their role in the management of GTPS.[50]

Injection Technique

The patient is placed in the lateral decubitus position on the contralateral hip, and the hips and knees are flexed in a comfortable position.[12,57,62] A high-frequency or medium-frequency linear-array transducer or low-frequency curvilinear-array transducer may be used depending on patient body habitus and desired field of view. The transducer is initially placed in the transverse plane over the lateral proximal femur. The transducer is then translated superiorly and the bony protuberance of the greater trochanter is identified. The apex of the greater trochanter is seen between the anterior and lateral facets (**Fig. 9**).[62] The gluteus minimus tendon is identified over the anterior facet and the gluteus medius tendon over the lateral facet. Evaluation should then be performed for subgluteus minimus and subgluteus medius bursal distention. The transducer is then moved posteriorly and the rounded posterior facet is identified posterior to the lateral facet. Greater trochanteric bursal distention may be identified between the gluteus maximus and posterior facet. The gluteus minimus and medius tendons and each trochanteric facet should be evaluated in both the transverse and longitudinal planes as indicated. When preprocedure scanning is

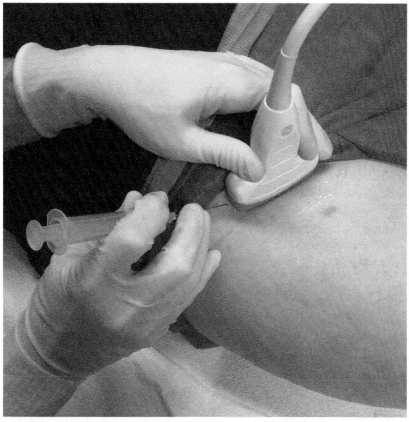

Fig. 6. Transverse oblique transducer and needle position parallel to the inguinal ligament for an in-plane iliopsoas bursa injection. (*Courtesy of* Mayo Foundation for Medical Education and Research, Rochester, MN; with permission.)

completed, the transducer is then again placed in the anatomic transverse plane over the greater trochanter (**Fig. 10**). The skin at the posterior edge of the transducer is marked with a marking pen and the area is prepped in the usual sterile manner. Following the delivery of local anesthesia, a 22-gauge 64-mm to 89-mm needle is advanced in-plane with the transducer using a posterior to anterior approach. The needle is then advanced under direct US guidance into the tissue plane between the superficial gluteus maximus-iliotibial band and the deep gluteus medius tendon, where the injectate is delivered (**Fig. 11**).

ULTRASOUND-GUIDED ISCHIAL BURSAL INJECTION
Diagnostic Criteria

The hamstring muscle complex consists of the semimembranosus, biceps femoris, and semitendinosus, which originate from the ischial tuberosity.[63,64] The semimembranosus originates on the superolateral aspect of the ischial tuberosity beneath the semitendinosus muscle and anterolateral to the conjoint tendon of the biceps femoris and semitendinosus. The semimembranosus tendon origin becomes aponeurotic soon after its origin and has the largest proximal tendon of the hamstring muscles.[64]

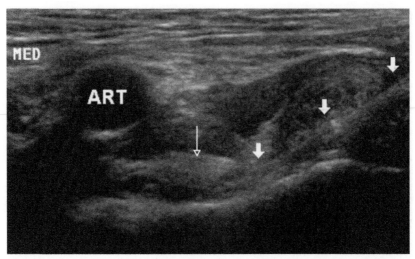

Fig. 7. US image of an in-plane iliopsoas bursa injection. The 3 solid arrows indicate the needle. The arrow with the open arrowhead indicates the iliopsoas tendon. ART, femoral artery; MED, medial. (*Courtesy of* Jay Smith, MD; with permission Mayo Foundation for Medical Education and Research, Rochester, MN.)

The ischial bursa is an inconstant (adventitial) bursa and, when not inflamed, is typically not visible on MRI or US.[65–67]

The differential diagnosis of gluteal region pain is broad and includes referred pain from the lumbar spine, sacroiliac joint disorders, piriformis syndrome, proximal hamstring tendinopathy, and ischial bursitis.[66,68,69] Inflammation of the ischial bursa most commonly occurs secondary to continuous and chronic irritation associated with sitting.[9,65–67,69] Ischial bursitis may also develop after a trauma to the buttocks or occur secondary to systemic inflammatory conditions such as systemic lupus erythematosus, ankylosing spondylitis, rheumatoid arthritis, or Reiter syndrome.[9,65,69] Ischial bursitis may present as a soft tissue mass, mimicking a tumor.[65,70,71] Patients with ischial bursitis most often experience pain in the buttocks and posterior thigh and, occasionally, in the lower leg that is worse with sitting and in the supine position.[9,72,73] Physical examination reveals tenderness to palpation over the ischial tuberosity.[67,72] Treatment options include oral analgesic or anti-inflammatory medications, avoidance of prolonged sitting, physical therapy to correct strength and flexibility deficits, and ice.[9,65,72] Diagnostic local anesthetic injections into the ischial bursa may be used when the diagnosis is uncertain. Corticosteroid injections have been performed for therapeutic purposes when other conservative treatments have been unsuccessful.[9,65,72]

A US-guided ischial bursa injection feasibility study and description of technique was performed by Wisniewski and colleagues[9] They performed cadaveric injections and demonstrated that US-guided ischial bursa injections can produce accurate ischial bursograms without overflow to adjacent structures or damage to surrounding neurovascular structures.[9] They also found that the sciatic nerve moves a significant distance laterally from the ischial tuberosity when the patient is in the lateral decubitus position with the hip flexed 90° in comparison with the prone position.[9] Therefore, placing the patient in the lateral decubitus position with the hip flexed 90° may decrease the risk of iatrogenic sciatic nerve injury during this procedure.[9]

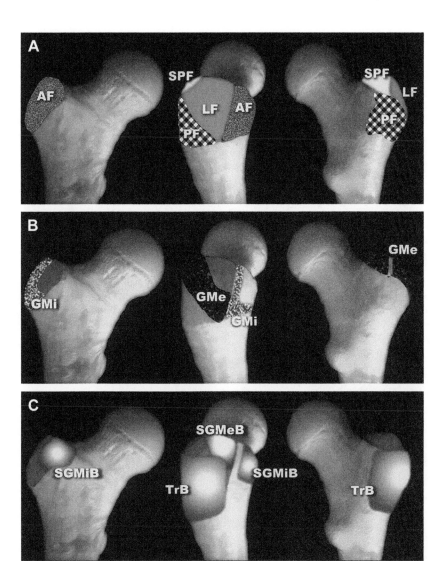

Fig. 8. (*A*) The proximal aspect of the femur in the anterior view (*left*), lateral view (*middle*), and posterior view (*right*) display the 4 facets of the greater trochanter: the anterior facet (AF), lateral facet (LF), posterior facet (PF), and superoposterior facet (SPF). (*B*) Osseous attachment sites of the gluteus medius (GMe) and gluteus minimus (GMi) tendons. (*C*) Locations of the bursae: trochanteric bursa (TrB), subgluteus medius bursa (SGMeB), and subgluteus minimus bursa (SGMiB). (*From* Pfirrmann CW, Chung CB, Theumann NH, et al. Greater trochanter of the hip: attachment of the abductor mechanism and a complex of three bursae-MR imaging and MR bursography in cadavers and MR imaging in asymptomatic volunteers. Radiology 2001;221:470; with permission.)

Injection Technique

The patient is placed in the lateral decubitus position on the contralateral hip, with the ipsilateral hip flexed 90°.[9] The ischial tuberosity is palpated and then the US transducer is placed in the transverse plane over the ischial tuberosity.[9]

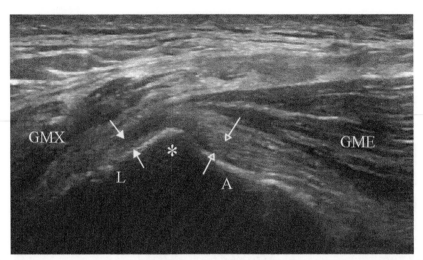

Fig. 9. Transverse US image over the greater trochanter demonstrating the bony apex (*asterisk*) between the gluteus medius (*arrows with solid arrowheads*) insertion on the lateral facet and the gluteus minimus (*arrows with open arrowheads*) insertion on the anterior facet. A, anterior facet; L, lateral facet; GME, gluteus medius muscle; GMX, gluteus maximus muscle. (*Courtesy of* Mayo Foundation for Medical Education and Research, Rochester, MN; with permission.)

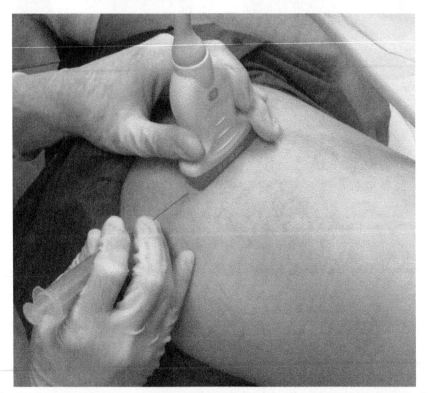

Fig. 10. Anatomic transverse transducer and needle position over the greater trochanter for an in-plane trochanteric bursa injection. (*Courtesy of* Mayo Foundation for Medical Education and Research, Rochester, MN; with permission.)

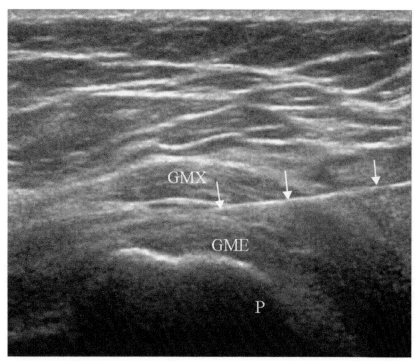

Fig. 11. US image of an in-plane trochanteric bursa injection. Arrows indicate needle. GME, gluteus medius tendon; GMX, gluteus maximus muscle; P, posterior facet. The right side of the image is posterior. (*Courtesy of* Jonathan T. Finnoff, DO; with permission Mayo Foundation for Medical Education and Research, Rochester, MN.)

A medium-frequency linear-array transducer or low-frequency curvilinear-array transducer may be used depending on patient body habitus and desired field of view. The transducer is then moved laterally and the sciatic nerve is identified superficial to the quadratus femoris muscle.[9] Following this, the transducer is positioned so that the gluteus maximus muscle, hamstring tendons, ischial tuberosity, and sciatic nerve are all visualized simultaneously (**Fig. 12**).[9] The skin at the lateral edge of the transducer is marked with a marking pen and the area is prepped in the usual sterile manner (**Fig. 13**). Following the delivery of local anesthesia, a 22-gauge 64-mm to 89-mm needle is advanced in-plane with the transducer from a lateral to medial approach. The needle is then advanced under direct US guidance into the region of the ischial bursa, located deep to the gluteus maximus and superficial to the hamstring tendons, and the injectate is delivered (**Fig. 14**).

ULTRASOUND-GUIDED PIRIFORMIS INJECTION
Diagnostic Criteria

The piriformis muscle lies deep to the gluteus maximus muscle and its primary function is to externally rotate the hip.[8,74–76] It passes through the greater sciatic foramen and inserts on the medial surface of the superior greater trochanter, and may merge with the tendons of the obturator internus and gemelli muscles.[77] The sciatic nerve typically exits the pelvic cavity through the inferior portion of the greater sciatic foramen deep to the piriformis. However, multiple anatomic variations of the nerve have

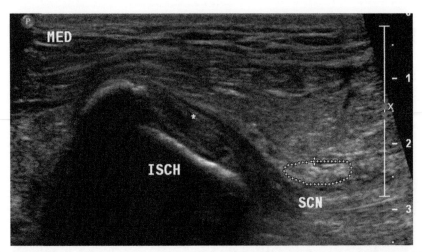

Fig. 12. US image demonstrating a short-axis view of the hamstring tendon origin (*asterisk*), ischium (ISCH), and sciatic nerve (SCN). The sciatic nerve is encircled. MED, medial. (*From* Wisniewski SJ, Hurdle MF, Erickson JM, et al. Ultrasound-guided ischial bursa injection: technique and positioning considerations. PM R 2014;6:58; with permission.)

been described. The undivided sciatic nerve may pass completely through the piriformis muscle or the nerve may divide, with the fibular division typically piercing the muscle and the tibial division traveling superiorly along the muscle.[75,77–79]

The symptoms of piriformis syndrome may vary and include pain in the low back, gluteal region, sacroiliac joint, and radicular leg pain.[75] It has been suggested that 6% to 8% of low back pain cases can be attributed to piriformis syndrome.[80] Piriformis syndrome often occurs after trauma to the buttocks.[74,77,81] Patients will often describe increased pain after sitting on the affected side.[77] Physical examination findings include tenderness over the piriformis muscle and pain with stretching of the piriformis muscle.[7,77,82] Piriformis syndrome is often a diagnosis of exclusion after other causes of buttock and lower limb pain have been eliminated.[8,75,76] Treatment options include stretching and strengthening exercises, physical modalities, oral analgesic or anti-inflammatory medications, and injections.[77,78,81]

Because piriformis syndrome is often a diagnosis of exclusion, a piriformis injection may be considered for diagnostic and/or therapeutic purposes. Piriformis injections, performed with local anesthetic, corticosteroid, and botulinum toxin type A, have been described.[74,83–86] Because of the deep location and small size of the piriformis muscle, and its close proximity to important neurovascular structures, image guidance has been recommended to improve safety and accuracy.[7] Piriformis injections have been described using fluoroscopy, US, CT scan, electromyography, and MRI guidance.[7,8,74,75,78,84,87,88]

Finnoff and colleagues[7] evaluated the accuracy of US-guided versus fluoroscopy-guided contrast-controlled piriformis injections in cadavers and found US-guided injections to be significantly more accurate (95%) than the fluoroscopy-guided injections (30%). A study by Fowler and colleagues[11] found no statistically significant difference in numeric pain scores, patient satisfaction, overall procedure time, or most functional outcomes when comparing US-guided versus fluoroscopy-guided with nerve-stimulation piriformis muscle local anesthetic and corticosteroid injections.

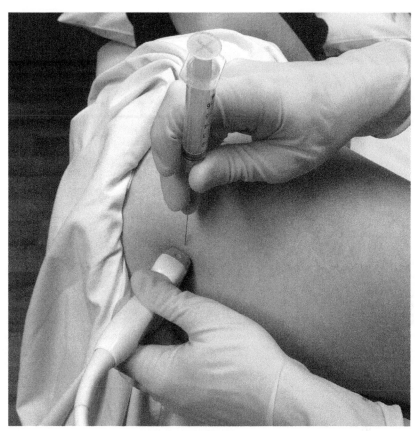

Fig. 13. Anatomic transverse transducer and needle position over the ischial tuberosity for an in-plane, lateral to medial ischial bursa injection. The subject is side-lying with the hip flexed to approximately 90°. (*Courtesy of* Mayo Foundation for Medical Education and Research, Rochester, MN; with permission.)

Injection Technique

With the patient in the prone position, the buttock region is scanned with a medium-frequency linear-array transducer or a low-frequency curvilinear-array transducer depending on body habitus and the desired field of view. The transducer is placed in the anatomic axial plane over the posterior superior iliac spine (PIIS).[8] The transducer is then moved inferiorly until the lateral sacrum is visualized medially and the PIIS is visualized laterally. The transducer is then moved inferior to the PIIS and the ilium will disappear from view, indicating the beginning of the greater sciatic notch.[7] The piriformis muscle is identified traversing from cephalomedial to caudolateral, deep to the overlying gluteus maximus muscle (**Fig. 15**).[8] In this orientation, the transducer is parallel to the course of the piriformis muscle. The piriformis muscle should be evaluated in both longitudinal and transverse views. Passive internal and external rotation of the hip can assist in identifying the piriformis muscle as it moves relative to the gluteus maximus (Video 3).[7,8,75] The sciatic nerve should then be identified and will most often be located deep to the piriformis muscle. Anatomic variations of the sciatic nerve course should be noted because it may necessitate adjustment in injection

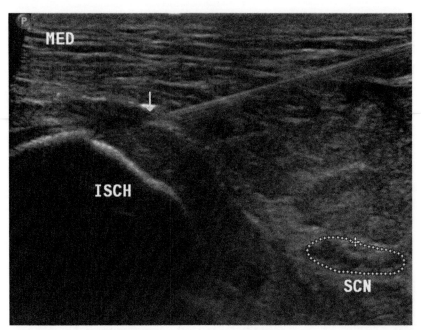

Fig. 14. US image demonstrating a needle within the ischial bursa. The gluteus maximus muscle is above the needle tip (*arrow*) and the hamstring tendon origin is below the needle tip. ISCH, ischium; MED, medial; SCN, sciatic nerve. (*From* Wisniewski SJ, Hurdle MF, Erickson JM, et al. Ultrasound-guided ischial bursa injection: technique and positioning considerations. PM R 2014;6:58; with permission.)

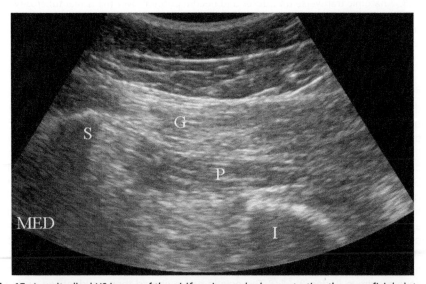

Fig. 15. Longitudinal US image of the piriformis muscle demonstrating the superficial gluteus maximus muscle (*G*) and piriformis muscle (*P*). I, ischium; MED, medial; S, sacrum. (*Courtesy of* Mayo Foundation for Medical Education and Research, Rochester, MN; with permission.)

technique and needle trajectory. The transducer is again placed in a cephalomedial to caudolateral orientation parallel to the piriformis muscle (**Fig. 16**). The skin at the lateral edge of the transducer is marked with a marking pen and the area is prepped in the usual sterile manner. Following the delivery of local anesthesia, a 22-gauge 89-mm needle is advanced in-plane with the transducer from a lateral to medial approach. The needle is then advanced under direct US guidance through the subcutaneous tissue and gluteus maximus until the piriformis muscle is entered, and the injectate is delivered (**Fig. 17**).

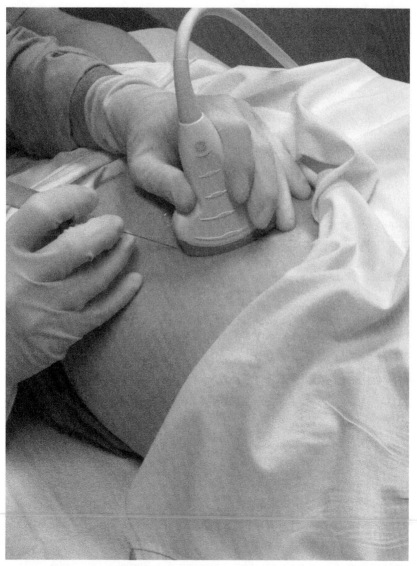

Fig. 16. US transducer and needle position over the piriformis muscle for an in-plane piriformis injection. Top of the picture is caudal and left side of the picture is lateral. (*Courtesy of* Mayo Foundation for Medical Education and Research, Rochester, MN; with permission.)

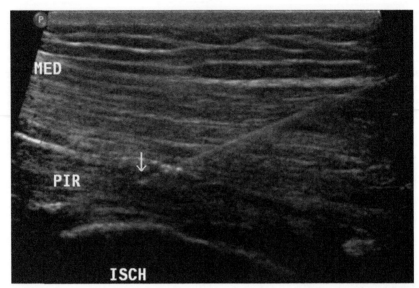

Fig. 17. US image demonstrating a needle placed within the piriformis muscle. Arrow indicates needle tip. ISCH, ischium; MED, medial; PIR, piriformis muscle. (*Courtesy of* Steve J. Wisniewski, MD; with permission Mayo Foundation for Medical Education and Research, Rochester, MN.)

SUMMARY

A variety of image-guided injections can be performed in the evaluation and treatment of hip pain. US confers many advantages compared with other commonly used imaging modalities, including real-time visualization of muscle, tendon, important neurovascular structures, and the needle during an intervention. US-guided injection techniques have been described for many commonly performed procedures in the hip region, and many studies have been performed demonstrating the safety and accuracy of these techniques. US guidance is, therefore, a highly recommended tool when performing procedures in the hip region.

SUPPLEMENTARY DATA

Supplementary data related to this article can be found at http://dx.doi.org/10.1016/j.pmr.2016.04.004.

REFERENCES

1. Tibor LM, Sekiya JK. Differential diagnosis of pain around the hip joint. Arthroscopy 2008;24:1407–21.
2. Jacobson JA, Bedi A, Sekiya JK, et al. Evaluation of the painful athletic hip: imaging options and imaging-guided injections. AJR Am J Roentgenol 2012; 199:516–24.
3. Guillin R, Cardinal E, Bureau NJ. Sonographic anatomy and dynamic study of the normal iliopsoas musculotendinous junction. Eur Radiol 2009;19:995–1001.
4. Jacobson JA, Khoury V, Brandon CJ. Ultrasound of the groin: techniques, pathology, and pitfalls. AJR Am J Roentgenol 2015;205:513–23.

5. Nestorova R, Violeta V, Tzvetanka P, et al. Ultrasonography of the hip. Med Ultrason 2012;14:217–24.
6. Smith J, Hurdle MF. Office-based ultrasound-guided intra-articular hip injection: technique for physiatric practice. Arch Phys Med Rehabil 2006;87:296–8.
7. Finnoff JT, Hurdle MF, Smith J. Accuracy of ultrasound-guided versus fluoroscopically guided contrast-controlled piriformis injections: a cadaveric study. J Ultrasound Med 2008;27:1157–63.
8. Smith J, Hurdle MF, Locketz AJ. Ultrasound-guided piriformis injection: technique description and verification. Arch Phys Med Rehabil 2006;87:1664–7.
9. Wisniewski SJ, Hurdle MF, Erickson JM, et al. Ultrasound-guided ischial bursa injection: technique and positioning considerations. PM R 2014;6:56–60.
10. Levi DS. Intra-articular hip injections using ultrasound guidance: accuracy using a linear array transducer. PM R 2013;5:129–34.
11. Fowler IM, Tucker AA, Weimerskirch BP. A randomized comparison of the efficacy of 2 techniques for piriformis muscle injection: ultrasound-guided versus nerve stimulator with fluoroscopic guidance. Reg Anesth Pain Med 2014;39:126–32.
12. McEvoy JR, Lee KS, Blankenbaker DG, et al. Ultrasound-guided corticosteroid injections for treatment of greater trochanteric pain syndrome: greater trochanter bursa versus subgluteus medius bursa. AJR Am J Roentgenol 2013;201:W313–7.
13. Rowbotham EL, Grainger AJ. Ultrasound-guided intervention around the hip joint. AJR Am J Roentgenol 2011;197:W122–7.
14. Yoong P, Guirguis R, Darrah R, et al. Evaluation of ultrasound-guided diagnostic local anaesthetic hip joint injection for osteoarthritis. Skeletal Radiol 2012;41: 981–5.
15. Odoom JE, Allen GM, Wilson DJ. Response to local anaesthetic injection as a predictor of successful hip surgery. Clin Radiol 1999;54:430–3.
16. Zhang W, Moskowitz RW, Nuki G, et al. OARSI recommendations for the management of hip and knee osteoarthritis, Part II: OARSI evidence-based, expert consensus guidelines. Osteoarthritis Cartilage 2008;16:137–62.
17. Robinson P, Keenan AM, Conaghan PG. Clinical effectiveness and dose response of image-guided intra-articular corticosteroid injection for hip osteoarthritis. Rheumatology 2007;46:285–91.
18. Pourbagher MA, Ozalay M, Pourbagher A. Accuracy and outcome of sonographically guided intra-articular sodium hyaluronate injections in patients with osteoarthritis of the hip. J Ultrasound Med 2005;24:1391–5.
19. Migliore A, Tormenta S, Lagana B. Safety of intra-articular hip injection of hyaluronic acid products by ultrasound guidance: an open study from ANTIAGE register. Eur Rev Med Pharmacol Sci 2013;17:1752–9.
20. Leopold SS, Battista V, Oliverio JA. Safety and efficacy of intraarticular hip injection using anatomic landmarks. Clin Orthop Relat Res 2001;391:192–7.
21. Masoud MA, Said HG. Intra-articular hip injection using anatomic surface landmarks. Arthrosc Tech 2013;2:e147–9.
22. Mei-Dan O, McConkey MO, Petersen B, et al. The anterior approach for a non-image-guided intra-articular hip injection. Arthroscopy 2013;29:1025–33.
23. Byrd JW, Potts EA, Allison RK, et al. Ultrasound-guided hip injections: a comparative study with fluoroscopy-guided injections. Arthroscopy 2014;30:42–6.
24. Kullenberg B, Runesson R, Tuvhag R, et al. Intraarticular corticosteroid injection: pain relief in osteoarthritis of the hip? J Rheumatol 2004;31:2265–8.
25. Santos-Ocampo AS, Santos-Ocampo RS. Non-contrast computed tomography-guided intra-articular corticosteroid injections of severe bilateral hip arthritis in a patient with ankylosing spondylitis. Clin Exp Rheumatol 2003;21:239–40.

26. Smith J, Hurdle MF, Weingarten TN. Accuracy of sonographically guided intra-articular injections in the native adult hip. J Ultrasound Med 2009;28:329–35.

27. Micu MC, Bogdan GD, Fodor D. Steroid injection for hip osteoarthritis: efficacy under ultrasound guidance. Rheumatology 2010;49:1490–4.

28. Sofka CM, Saboeiro G, Adler RS. Ultrasound-guided adult hip injections. J Vasc Inverv Radiol 2005;16:1121–3.

29. Kantarci F, Ozbayrak M, Gulsen F, et al. Ultrasound-guided injection for MR arthrography of the hip: comparison of two different techniques. Skeletal Radiol 2013;42:37–42.

30. Hoeber S, Aly AR, Ashworth N, et al. Ultrasound-guided hip joint injections are more accurate than landmark-guided injections: a systematic review and meta-analysis. Br J Sports Med 2016;50(7):392–6.

31. Finnoff JT, Hall MM, Adams E, et al. American Medical Society for Sports Medicine (AMSSM) position statement: interventional musculoskeletal ultrasound in sports medicine. PM R 2015;7:151–68.

32. Atchia I, Kane D, Reed MR, et al. Efficacy of a single ultrasound-guided injection for the treatment of hip osteoarthritis. Ann Rheum Dis 2011;70:110–6.

33. Furtado RN, Pereira DF, da Luz KR, et al. Effectiveness of imaging-guided intra-articular injection: a comparison study between fluoroscopy and ultrasound. Rev Bras Rheumatol 2013;53:476–82.

34. Robben SG, Lequin MH, Diepstraten AF, et al. Anterior joint capsule of the normal hip and in children with transient synovitis: US study with anatomic and histologic correlation. Radiology 1999;210:499–507.

35. Sofka CM, Adler RS, Danon MA. Sonography of the acetabular labrum: visualization of labral injuries during intra-articular injections. J Ultrasound Med 2006;25:1321–6.

36. Blankenbaker DG, Tuite MJ. Iliopsoas musculotendinous unit. Semin Musculoskelet Radiol 2008;12:13–27.

37. Polster JM, Elgabaly M, Lee H, et al. MRI and gross anatomy of the iliopsoas tendon complex. Skeletal Radiol 2008;37:55–8.

38. Dauffenbach J, Pingree MJ, Wisniewski SJ, et al. Distribution pattern of sonographically guided iliopsoas injections: cadaveric investigation using coned beam computed tomography. J Ultrasound Med 2014;33:405–14.

39. Idjadi J, Meislin R. Symptomatic snapping hip: targeted treatment for maximum pain relief. Phys Sportsmed 2004;32:25–31.

40. Brew CJ, Stockley I, Grainger AJ, et al. Iliopsoas tendonitis caused by overhang of a collared femoral prosthesis. J Arthroplasty 2011;504:e17–9.

41. Tormenta S, Sconfienza LM, Iannessi F, et al. Prevalence study of iliopsoas bursitis in a cohort of 860 patients affected by symptomatic hip osteoarthritis. Ultrasound Med Biol 2012;38:1352–6.

42. Agten CA, Rosskopf AB, Zingg PO, et al. Outcomes after fluoroscopically guided iliopsoas bursa injection for suspected iliopsoas tendinopathy. Eur Radiol 2015;25:865–71.

43. Nunley RM, Wilson JM, Gilula L, et al. Iliopsoas bursa injections can be beneficial for pain after total hip arthroplasty. Clin Orthop Relat Res 2010;468:519–26.

44. Blankenbaker DG, De Smet AA, Keene JS. Sonography of the iliopsoas tendon and injection of the iliopsoas bursa for diagnosis and management of the painful snapping hip. Skeletal Radiol 2006;35:565–71.

45. Wank R, Miller TT, Shapiro JF. Sonographically guided injection of anesthetic for iliopsoas tendinopathy after total hip arthroplasty. J Clin Ultrasound 2004;32: 354–7.
46. Adler RS, Buly R, Ambrose R, et al. Diagnostic and therapeutic use of sonography-guided iliopsoas peritendinous injections. AJR Am J Roentgenol 2005;185:940–3.
47. Strauss EJ, Nho SJ, Kelly BT. Greater trochanteric pain syndrome. Sports Med Arthrosc 2010;18:113–9.
48. Pfirrmann CW, Chung CB, Theumann NH, et al. Greater trochanter of the hip: attachment of the abductor mechanism and a complex of three bursae-MR imaging and MR bursography in cadavers and MR imaging in asymptomatic volunteers. Radiology 2001;221:469–77.
49. Dwek J, Pfirrmann C, Stanley A, et al. MR imaging of the hip abductors: normal anatomy and commonly encountered pathology at the greater trochanter. Magn Reson Imaging Clin N Am 2005;13:691–704.
50. Mallow M, Nazarian LN. Greater trochanteric pain syndrome diagnosis and treatment. Phys Med Rehabil Clin N Am 2014;25:279–89.
51. Robertson WJ, Gardner MJ, Barker JU, et al. Anatomy and dimensions of the gluteus medius tendon insertion. Arthroscopy 2008;24:130–6.
52. Williams BS, Cohen SP. Greater trochanteric pain syndrome: a review of anatomy, diagnosis, and treatment. Anesth Analg 2009;108:1662–70.
53. Segal NA, Felson DT, Torner JC, et al. Greater trochanteric pain syndrome: epidemiology and associated factors. Arch Phys Med Rehabil 2007;88:988–92.
54. Fearon AM, Cook JL, Scarvell JM, et al. Greater trochanteric pain syndrome negatively affects work, physical activity and quality of life: a case control study. J Arthroplasty 2014;29:383–6.
55. Dunn T, Heller CA, McCarthy SW, et al. Anatomical study of the "trochanteric bursa". Clin Anat 2003;16:233–40.
56. Silva F, Adams T, Feinstein J, et al. Trochanteric bursitis: refuting the myth of inflammation. J Clin Rheumatol 2008;14:82–6.
57. Labrosse JM, Cardinal E, Leduc BE, et al. Effectiveness of ultrasound-guided corticosteroid injection for the treatment of gluteus medius tendinopathy. AJR Am J Roentgenol 2010;194:202–6.
58. Shbeeb MI, O'Duffy JD, Michet CJ, et al. Evaluation of glucocorticosteroid injection for the treatment of trochanteric bursitis. J Rheumatol 1996;23:2104–6.
59. Cohen SP, Narvaez JC, Lebovits AH, et al. Corticosteroid injections for trochanteric bursitis: is fluoroscopy necessary? A pilot study. Br J Anaesth 2005;94: 100–6.
60. Finnoff JT, Fowler SP, Lai JK, et al. Treatment of chronic tendinopathy with ultrasound-guided needle tenotomy and platelet-rich plasma injection. PM R 2011;3:900–11.
61. Jacobson JA, Rubin J, Yablon CM, et al. Ultrasound-guided fenestration of tendons about the hip and pelvis: clinical outcomes. J Ultrasound Med 2015;34: 2029–35.
62. Peng PW. Ultrasound-guided interventional procedures in pain medicine: a review of anatomy, sonoanatomy, and procedures. Part IV: hip. Reg Anesth Pain Med 2013;38:264–73.
63. Koulouris G, Connell D. Hamstring muscle complex: an imaging review. Radiographics 2005;25:571–86.
64. Linklater JM, Hamilton B, Carmichael J, et al. Hamstring injuries: anatomy, imaging, and intervention. Semin Musculoskelet Radiol 2010;14:131–61.

65. Van Miegham IM, Boets A, Sciot R, et al. Ischiogluteal bursitis: an uncommon type of bursitis. Skeletal Radiol 2005;33:413–6.

66. Hitora T, Kawaguchi Y, Masaki M, et al. Ischiogluteal bursitis: a report of three cases with MR findings. Rheumatol Int 2009;29:455–8.

67. Ekiz T, Bicici V, Hatioglu C, et al. Ischial pain and sitting disability due to ischio-gluteal bursitis: visual vignette. Pain Physician 2015;18:E657–9.

68. Ripani M, Continenza MA, Cacchio A, et al. The ischiatic region: normal and MRI anatomy. J Sports Med Phys Fitness 2006;46:468–75.

69. Kim SM, Shin MJ, Kim KS, et al. Imaging features of ischial bursitis with an emphasis on ultrasonography. Skeletal Radiol 2002;31:631–6.

70. Volk M, Gmeinsieser J, Hanika H, et al. Ischiogluteal bursitis mimicking soft-tissue metastasis from a renal cell carcinoma. Eur Radiol 1998;8:1140–1.

71. Toshihiro A, Yamamoto T, Marui T, et al. Ischiogluteal bursitis: multimodality imaging findings. Clin Orthop Relat Res 2003;406:214–7.

72. Mills GM, Baethge BA. Ischiogluteal bursitis in cancer patients: an infrequently recognized cause of pain. Am J Clin Oncol 1993;16:229–31.

73. Choo KH, Lee SM, Lee YH, et al. Non-infectious ischiogluteal bursitis: MRI find-ings. Korean J Radiol 2004;5:280–6.

74. Ozisik PA, Toru M, Denk CC, et al. CT-guided piriformis muscle injection for the treatment of piriformis syndrome. Turk Neurosurg 2014;24:471–7.

75. Fabregat G, Rosello M, Asensio-Samper JM, et al. Computer-tomographic verifi-cation of ultrasound-guided piriformis muscle injection: a feasibility study. Pain Physician 2014;17:507–13.

76. Michel F, Decavel P, Toussirot E, et al. The piriformis muscle syndrome: an explo-ration of anatomical context, pathophysiological hypotheses and diagnostic criteria. Ann Phys Rehabil Med 2013;56:300–11.

77. Boyajian-O'Neill LA, McClain RL, Coleman MK, et al. Diagnosis and management of piriformis syndrome: an osteopathic approach. J Am Osteopath Assoc 2008; 108:657–64.

78. Gonzalez P, Pepper M, Sullivan W, et al. Confirmation of needle placement within the piriformis muscle of a cadaveric specimen using anatomic landmarks and fluoroscopic guidance. Pain Physician 2008;11:327–31.

79. Al-Al-Shaikh M, Michel F, Parratte B, et al. An MRI evaluation of changes in piriformis muscle morphology induced by botulinum toxin injections in the treat-ment of piriformis syndrome. Diagn Interv Imaging 2015;96:37–43.

80. Halin R. Sciatic pain and the piriformis muscle. Postgrad Med 1983;74:69–72.

81. Windisch G, Braun EM, Anderhuber F. Piriformis muscle: clinical anatomy and consideration of the piriformis syndrome. Surg Radilo Anat 2007;29:37–45.

82. Cass SP. Piriformis syndrome: a cause of nondiscogenic sciatica. Curr Sports Med Rep 2015;14:41–4.

83. Misirlioglu TO, Akgun K, Palamar D, et al. Piriformis syndrome: comparison of the effectiveness of local anesthetic and corticosteroid injections: a double-blinded, randomized controlled study. Pain Physician 2015;18:163–71.

84. Blunk JM, Nowotny M, Scharf J, et al. MRI verification of ultrasound-guided infiltrations of local anesthetics into the piriformis muscle. Pain Med 2013;14: 1593–9.

85. Santamato A, Micello MF, Valeno G, et al. Ultrasound-guided injection of botuli-num toxin Type A for piriformis muscle syndrome: a case report and review of the literature. Toxins 2015;7:3045–56.

86. Jeong HS, Lee GY, Lee EG, et al. Long-term assessment of clinical outcomes of ultrasound-guided steroid injections in patients with piriformis syndrome. Ultrasonography 2015;34:206–10.
87. Filler A, Haynes J, Jordan S, et al. Sciatica of nondisc origin and piriformis syndrome: diagnosis by magnetic resonance neurography and interventional magnetic resonance imaging with outcome of resulting treatment. J Neurosurg Spine 2005;2:99–115.
88. Betts A. Combined fluoroscopic and nerve stimulator technique for injection of the piriformis muscle. Pain Physician 2004;7:279–81.

Ultrasound-Guided Knee Procedures

Daniel R. Lueders, MD[a], Jay Smith, MD[a,b,c], Jacob L. Sellon, MD[a,*]

KEYWORDS

- Injection • Knee • Musculoskeletal • Sonography • Sports Ultrasound • Ultrasound
- Ultrasound-guided injection

KEY POINTS

- The anatomy of the knee is particularly amenable to ultrasound imaging, and therefore most knee structures can be accurately targeted using ultrasound guidance.
- Studies of ultrasound-guided knee procedures have consistently shown high accuracy.
- Using ultrasound guidance for knee procedures is particularly useful for obese patients, diagnostic injection specificity, safety around neurovascular structures, and precise targeting of pathology.
- More studies are needed to assess the clinical efficacy and cost-effectiveness of various ultrasound-guided knee procedures.

INTRODUCTION

The anatomy of the knee is particularly amenable to ultrasound (US) imaging, and therefore most knee structures can be accurately targeted using US guidance. In most individuals, these structures are superficial, and the overlying soft tissues are mobile and compressible, facilitating excellent visualization with a high-frequency linear array transducer. The circumferential accessibility to the knee affords flexibility and often multiple procedural approach options. In most cases, an in-plane approach (ie, parallel to the transducer) can be easily achieved, improving needle visualization and injection safety.

ULTRASOUND-GUIDED KNEE JOINT INJECTIONS
Indications

General indications for US-guided (USG) knee joint injections include failure of a prior landmark-guided (LG) knee joint injection, complex postoperative or

Disclosure: The authors have nothing to disclose.
[a] Department of Physical Medicine and Rehabilitation, Mayo Clinic Sports Medicine Center, Mayo Clinic, 200 1st St Southwest, Rochester, MN 55905, USA; [b] Department of Radiology, Mayo Clinic, 200 1st St SW, Rochester, MN 55905, USA; [c] Department of Anatomy, Mayo Clinic, 200 1st St SW, Rochester, MN 55905, USA
* Corresponding author.
E-mail address: sellon.jacob@mayo.edu

Phys Med Rehabil Clin N Am 27 (2016) 631–648
http://dx.doi.org/10.1016/j.pmr.2016.04.010
1047-9651/16/$ – see front matter © 2016 Elsevier Inc. All rights reserved.

posttraumatic anatomy, obese body habitus, need for diagnostic specificity, and orthobiologic injections (eg, hyaluronic acid, platelet-rich plasma, bone marrow aspirate concentrate), in which intra-articular placement is essential for the treatment mechanism.[1–4]

Cost-Effectiveness

- Although studies have generally shown superior accuracy of USG knee joint[2,3] injections, there remains some debate regarding cost-effectiveness.
- Sibbitt and colleagues[5] showed that, relative to LG knee joint corticosteroid injections, USG injections led to 13% reduction ($17) in cost per patient per year and 58% ($224) reduction in cost per responder per year.
- Because injection accuracy is likely more critical for orthobiologic versus corticosteroid injection efficacy, USG may be more cost-effective when delivering orthobiologic injections, although this has not been specifically investigated.

KNEE JOINT INJECTION: SUPRAPATELLAR APPROACH
Indications

- Easy access to the joint via the suprapatellar recess.[1,2,4,5]
- Avoid contact with cartilage and other intra-articular structures.
- Preferred approach for visualizing and aspirating effusion.

Accuracy

- Bum and colleagues[4] showed greater accuracy with the suprapatellar USG approach (96.0%) than LG injections (83.7%).
- Curtiss and colleagues[2] showed 100% accuracy with the suprapatellar USG approach across experience levels, whereas LG injections showed less accuracy and more variability (55%–100%).

Safety

There are no published complications with this approach.

Clinical Efficacy

Relative to LG injections, the suprapatellar USG approach resulted in 48% reduction in procedural pain, 42% reduction in pain at outcome, and 36% increase in therapeutic duration.[5]

Positioning

- Patient supine with knee partially flexed (**Fig. 1**A).
- Transducer in anatomic transverse plane over suprapatellar recess.

Preprocedural Scan

- Visualize suprapatellar recess deep to the quadriceps fat pad/tendon and superficial to the prefemoral fat pad.
- If effusion present, this makes for an effective target (**Fig. 1**B). Small effusions can be enhanced with knee flexion. Check dependent portions of joint recess.
- Note depth of target for planning skin entry point.

Needle Approach

- In plane relative to transducer (**Fig. 1**C, D).
- Advance lateral to medial or medial to lateral.

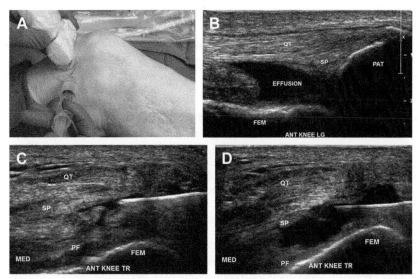

Fig. 1. (*A*) Setup for a right knee sonographically guided, lateral-to-medial, suprapatellar joint recess injection. Proximal is left. (*B*) Sonographic longitudinal view of an effusion in the suprapatellar joint recess between the suprapatellar fat pad and quadriceps tendon. Note that this is a different orientation from that depicted in **Fig. 1**A. (*C*) Sonographic transverse view of a lateral-to-medial injection, in plane with the transducer into the suprapatellar joint recess between the suprapatellar fat pad and prefemoral fat pad. Medial is left. (*D*) Injectate distending the suprapatellar joint recess. Medial is left. ANT, anterior, FEM, femur, LG, longitudinal; MED, medial; PAT, patella; PF, prefemoral fat pad, QT, quadriceps tendon, SP, suprapatellar fat pad, TR, transverse.

Pearls

- To confirm plane of suprapatellar recess, use external pressure to mobilize prefemoral fat pad and visualize differential motion relative to quadriceps tendon.
- Do not confuse hypoechoic fat pad or synovitis with an effusion; the latter is typically compressible and displaceable.
- During injection, confirm injectate flow distally into patellofemoral joint by visualizing suprapatellar recess in anatomic sagittal plane.

KNEE JOINT INJECTION: PATELLOFEMORAL APPROACH
Indications

No effusion present and/or suprapatellar recess is difficult to visualize.[1,3]

Accuracy

Ninety-five percent using lateral patellofemoral approach (out of plane, or perpendicular, relative to transducer), but there have been no direct comparisons with other USG approaches or LG injections.[3]

Safety

No published complications with this approach.

Clinical Efficacy

No published studies have evaluated the clinical efficacy of this approach.

Positioning

- Patient supine with knee extended (**Fig. 2**A).
- Transducer in anatomic axial plane over the anterolateral knee with visualization of the lateral patella and lateral femoral epicondyle.
- Positioning is similar on the medial side for a medial patellofemoral approach.

Preprocedural Scan

- Lateral (or medial) patellofemoral recess adjacent to patellofemoral joint.
- Check dependent regions of recess for small effusion.

Needle Approach

- Out of plane: advance proximal to distal or distal to proximal (**Fig. 2**B).
  - Use walk-down technique until needle descends into patellofemoral joint.
- In plane: advance lateral to medial or medial to lateral (**Fig. 2**C).
  - Can inject into patellofemoral recess or directly into patellofemoral joint.

Pearls

- If no effusion to target in joint recess, it is essential to visualize needle tip pass deep to patellofemoral retinaculum and periretinacular tissue before injecting.
- During injection, confirm intra-articular flow by visualizing injectate flow into suprapatellar recess.

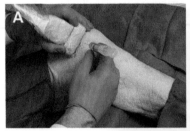
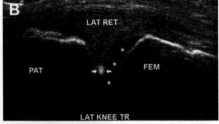
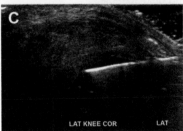

Fig. 2. (*A*) Setup for a right knee sonographically guided lateral patellofemoral joint injection, out of plane with the transducer. Proximal is left. (*B*) Sonographic oblique transverse view of the lateral patellofemoral joint space deep to the lateral patellofemoral retinaculum between the patella and femur showing an injection out of plane with the transducer. Arrows identify the needle tip in short axis adjacent to the femoral articular cartilage (asterisks). (*C*) Sonographic coronal view of lateral patellofemoral joint space injection in plane with the transducer. Right is lateral/distal. Note this is a different orientation than that depicted in **Fig. 2**A. COR, coronal; LAT, lateral; LAT RET, lateral patellofemoral retinaculum.

KNEE JOINT INJECTION: POSTEROMEDIAL APPROACH
Indications

- No effusion present and/or suprapatellar recess is difficult to visualize.[1,6]
- Patellofemoral osteoarthritis limits patellofemoral approach.
- Performing Baker cyst aspiration in conjunction with knee joint injection (allows for single sterile preparation without changing patient position).

Accuracy

- One study showed 100% accuracy of this approach, but made no direct comparisons with other USG approaches or LG injections.[6]

Safety

No complications with this approach in the series mentioned earlier (n = 67).[6]

Clinical Efficacy

No published studies have evaluated the clinical efficacy of this approach.

Positioning

- Patient prone with knee extended (**Fig. 3**A).
- Transducer in anatomic axial plane over the posteromedial femoral condyle.

Preprocedural Scan

- Identify chondral surface of posteromedial femoral condyle.
- Identify and avoid popliteal neurovascular bundle and saphenous nerve.

Needle Approach

In plane: advance medial to lateral between semimembranosus (SM) and gracilis just superficial to articular surface of medial femoral condyle (**Fig. 3**B).

Pearls

During injection, confirm intra-articular flow along superficial surface of hypoechoic medial femoral condyle cartilage.

BAKER CYST ASPIRATION/FENESTRATION
Indications

- Complete aspiration of cyst, including multilocular cysts.[1,7,8]

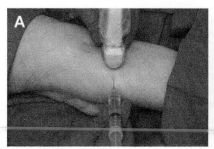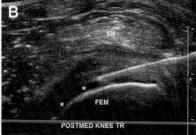

Fig. 3. (A) Setup for a right knee sonographically guided posteromedial knee joint injection, in plane with the transducer. Proximal is left, posterior is top. (B) Sonographic transverse view of a posteromedial-to-lateral knee joint injection, in plane with the transducer, and deep to semimembranosus (SM) and gently contacting the posterior medial femoral condyle articular cartilage (*asterisk*). POSTMED, posteromedial.

- Avoid injury to popliteal neurovascular bundle.
- Targeting walls and/or stalk of cyst with fenestration.

Accuracy

No published studies have evaluated USG relative to LG popliteal cyst aspirations.

Safety

Smith and colleagues[8] reported no complications in a series of 47 USG Baker cyst aspiration, fenestration, and cortisone injection procedures.

Clinical Efficacy

Smith and colleagues[8] reported significant clinical improvement at a mean 90.2 weeks of follow-up after USG Baker cyst aspiration, fenestration, and cortisone injection procedures.

Positioning

- Patient prone with knee extended.
- Transducer in anatomic transverse (**Fig. 4**A) or sagittal (**Fig. 4**B) plane over dependent part of cyst.

Preprocedural Scan

- Identify and avoid popliteal neurovascular bundle.
- Confirm Baker cyst (vs tumor, aneurysm, or ganglion cyst) (**Fig. 4**C).
  - Anechoic, compressible cyst with stalk emanating from posteromedial knee joint between medial gastrocnemius and SM.
  - Do not mistake anisotropic tendon for cyst/fluid. Toggle the transducer to confirm, particularly for the SM tendon, which may appear round and hypoechoic in this region because of anisotropy.
  - Cyst may be simple, multiloculated, or ruptured. May have hyperechoic synovial debris.
  - Assess with Doppler. May see cyst wall hyperemia, but be wary of extensive hyperemia or flow within cyst, which may suggest a soft tissue mass.
  - If cyst is in atypical location or has atypical soft tissue features, further investigation (eg, MRI with and without intravenous contrast) may be warranted to evaluate for the presence of a soft tissue tumor before consideration of a procedure.

Needle Approach

In plane: advance medial to lateral (or lateral to medial) (**Fig. 4**D) or distal to proximal (**Fig. 4**E), depending on shape and orientation of cyst.

Pearls

- Fenestration more accurately performed if done before aspiration.
- Aspirate with needle tip in most dependent portion of cyst (in prone position).
- Consider addressing source of cyst fluid with intra-articular injection (eg, corticosteroid).[7]

ILIOTIBIAL BAND PERITENDINOUS INJECTION
Indications

- Diagnostic and/or therapeutic injection for pain attributed to iliotibial band (ITB) syndrome.[1,9]
- Avoid injury to the common fibular nerve.

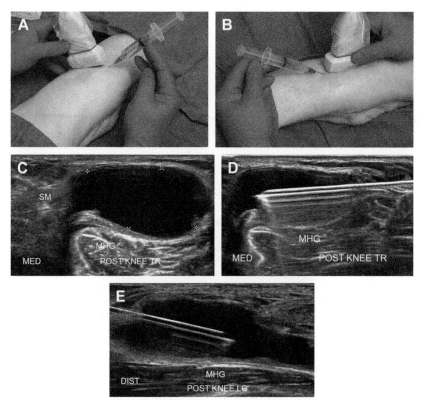

Fig. 4. (*A*) Setup for a right knee sonographically guided Baker cyst aspiration, in plane with the transducer and transverse to the leg. Proximal is bottom left, posterior is top. (*B*) Setup for a left knee sonographically guided Baker cyst injection, in plane with the transducer and longitudinal to the leg. Distal is left, posterior is top. (*C*) Sonographic transverse view of a Baker cyst (outlined by + and ×) between the SM tendon and medial head of gastrocnemius (MHG). (*D*) Sonographic transverse view of a lateral-to-medial Baker cyst aspiration, in plane with the transducer, between the SM tendon (SM) and MHG. (*E*) Sonographic longitudinal view of a distal-to-proximal Baker cyst aspiration, in plane with the transducer and superficial to the MHG. DIST, distal; MED, medial; POST, posterior.

Accuracy

No published studies have evaluated USG relative to LG ITB peritendinous injections.

Safety

No published complications with this injection.

Clinical Efficacy

No published studies have evaluated or compared the clinical efficacy of USG versus LG injections.

Positioning

- Patient is placed in lateral recumbent position with side to be injected facing up (**Fig. 5**A).
- Transducer in anatomic transverse plane over the ITB at the lateral femoral epicondyle.

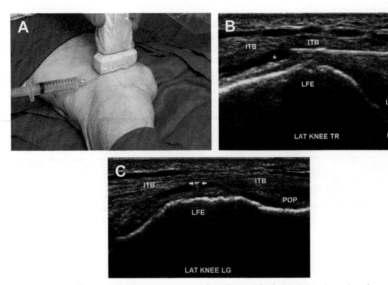

Fig. 5. (*A*) Setup for a right knee sonographically guided ITB injection, in plane with the transducer and in short axis to the ITB. Proximal is upper left, anterior is right. (*B*) Sonographic transverse view of a posterior-to-anterior injection, in plane with the transducer, between the ITB and the lateral femoral epicondyle (LFE). Note fluid (*asterisk*) deep to ITB. (C) Sonographic coronal/longitudinal view of a posterior-to-anterior injection, out of plane with the transducer, between the ITB and LFE (*arrows* denote needle tip). Popliteus is visualized on the distal, posterolateral femur. LG, lateral gastrocnemius; POP, popliteus.

Preprocedural Scan

- Confirm tendinopathic or tender region of distal ITB, most commonly at level of lateral femoral epicondyle.
- Identify and avoid common fibular nerve.

Needle Approach

In plane/Out of plane: advance posterior to anterior at the deep surface of the ITB (**Fig. 5**B, C).

Pearls

Float transducer to identify occult fluid deep to ITB. Be aware that what looks like fluid in the ITB bursa may be a knee effusion in the lateral joint recess.[9]

PES ANSERINE BURSA INJECTION
Indications

- Diagnostic and/or therapeutic injection for pain attributed to pes anserine tendinopathy/bursopathy.[1,10]
- Avoid injury to the inferior medial geniculate artery and saphenous nerve.

Accuracy

Finnoff and colleagues[10] showed accuracy rate of 92% using USG injections compared with 17% for LG injections.

Safety

No published complications with this injection.

Clinical Efficacy

No published studies have evaluated or compared the clinical efficacy of USG versus LG injections.

Positioning

- Patient supine with the hip externally rotated and knee slightly flexed (**Fig. 6**A)
- Transducer
  - Oblique coronal plane, long axis (LAX) to pes anserine tendons.
  - Coronal plane, oblique short axis (SAX) to tendons.

Preprocedural Scan

- Identify semitendinosus tendon in SAX in distal posteromedial thigh.
- Trace semitendinosus tendon distally/anteriorly as it converges with gracilis and sartorius tendons.
- As tendons are traced to anteromedial tibia, identify medial collateral ligament (MCL) passing deep to tendons.
- Pes anserine bursa is in plane deep to tendons and superficial to MCL.
- Identify and avoid inferior medial geniculate artery deep to MCL.
- Note saphenous nerve emerging superficial to gracilis and avoid during procedure.
- Identify and avoid great saphenous vein posterior to pes anserine tendons.

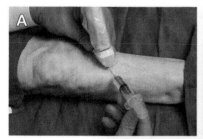
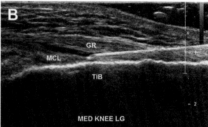
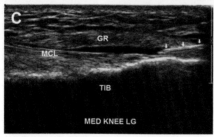

Fig. 6. (A) Setup for a right knee sonographically guided pes anserine bursa injection, long axis to the pes anserine tendons and in plane with the transducer. Proximal is left, medial is top. (B) Sonographic oblique longitudinal view of a distal/anterior to proximal/posterior pes anserine bursa injection, in plane with the transducer and long axis to the pes anserine tendons. The needle passes through the gracilis (GR) tendon, into the pes anserine bursa, which is superficial to the obliquely inserting medial collateral ligament (MCL) into the tibia. (C) Sonographic coronal/longitudinal view of a distal-to-proximal pes anserine bursa injection, in plane with the transducer, oblique short axis to the traversing gracilis (GR) tendon, and superficial to the MCL. The needle is denoted by arrows. Note this is a different orientation than that depicted in **Fig. 6**A. TIB, tibia.

Needle Approach

- In plane relative to transducer.
- LAX to tendons: advance distal/anterior to proximal/posterior (**Fig. 6**B).
- Oblique SAX to tendons: advance distal to proximal (**Fig. 6**C).

Pearls

Tilting the transducer can cause the tendons to appear anisotropic and facilitate differentiation from the underlying MCL.

SUPERFICIAL/DEEP INFRAPATELLAR BURSAE INJECTIONS
Indications

- Diagnostic and/or therapeutic injection for pain attributed to infrapatellar bursopathy.[1]
- Avoid intratendinous corticosteroid injection.

Accuracy

No published studies have evaluated or compared USG versus LG injections.

Safety

No published complications with these injections.

Clinical Efficacy

No published studies have evaluated or compared the clinical efficacy of USG versus LG for these injections.

Positioning

- Patient supine with the knee slightly flexed (**Fig. 7**A).
- Transducer in anatomic transverse plane over distal patellar tendon.

Preprocedural Scan

- Identify fluid superficial/deep to distal patellar tendon (**Fig. 7**B).
- Minimal fluid in deep infrapatellar bursa is physiologic.
- Excess fluid, presence of color or power Doppler flow, and sonopalpatory tenderness suggest bursitis.

Needle Approach

In plane/Out of plane: advance lateral to medial either deep (**Fig. 7**C, D) or superficial (**Fig. 7**E) to distal patellar tendon.

Pearls

- Float transducer to identify occult superficial infrapatellar bursal fluid.
- Sliding lateral/medial to midline patellar tendon can reveal dependent deep infrapatellar bursal fluid.

POPLITEUS TENDON SHEATH INJECTION
Indications

- Diagnostic and/or therapeutic injection for pain attributed to popliteus tendinopathy or snapping popliteus tendon.[1,11]
- Avoid common fibular nerve injury or intratendinous corticosteroid injection.

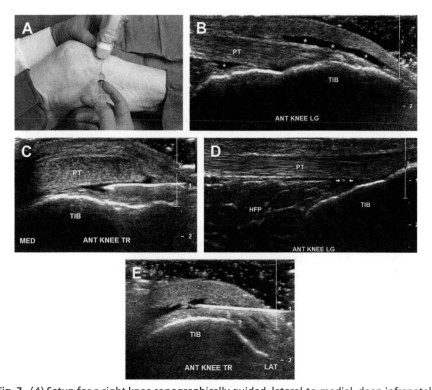

Fig. 7. (*A*) Setup for a right knee sonographically guided, lateral-to-medial, deep infrapatellar bursa injection, in plane with the transducer. A similar approach can be used to target the superficial infrapatellar bursa. Proximal is left. (*B*) Sonographic longitudinal view showing fluid (*asterisk*) within the superficial and deep infrapatellar bursae, superficial and deep to the patellar tendon near its insertion into tibia. (*C*) Sonographic transverse view of a lateral-to-medial injection, in plane with the transducer into the deep infrapatellar bursa, between the tibia and patellar tendon. (*D*) Sonographic longitudinal view of a lateral-to-medial injection, out of plane with the transducer, into the deep infrapatellar bursa. The needle tip is identified between the arrows. (*E*) Sonographic transverse view of a lateral-to-medial superficial infrapatellar bursa injection, in plane with the transducer. Needle tip is superficial to the patellar tendon near its insertion into the tibia. HFP, Hoffa fat pad; PT, patellar tendon.

Accuracy

- Smith and colleagues[11] showed 100% accuracy with LAX approach and 83% accuracy with SAX approach.
- No published studies have compared USG with LG injections.

Safety

No published complications with this injection.

Clinical Efficacy

No published studies have evaluated or compared the clinical efficacy of USG versus LG injections.

Positioning

- Patient lateral recumbent with the top/symptomatic knee slightly flexed and leg internally rotated.
- Transducer:
  - Anatomic oblique coronal plane (proximal end anterior) over posterior aspect of the lateral femoral epicondyle, LAX to popliteus tendon (**Fig. 8A**).
  - Anatomic oblique coronal plane (proximal end posterior) over lateral knee, SAX to the popliteus tendon (**Fig. 8B**).

Preprocedural Scan

- Place proximal end of transducer on lateral femoral epicondyle and visualize fibular collateral ligament (FCL) and popliteus sulcus with popliteus in oblique transverse view.
- Approach LAX to tendon:
  - Keeping popliteus tendon fibers in view, rotate distal end of transducer posteriorly until popliteus tendon is visualized in LAX.
- Approach SAX to tendon:
  - Keeping popliteus tendon fibers in view, rotate proximal end of transducer posteriorly until popliteus tendon is visualized in SAX.
- Identify and avoid common fibular nerve.

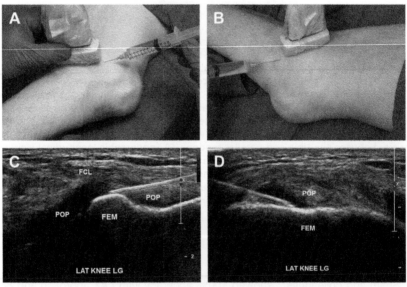

Fig. 8. (*A*) Setup for a right knee sonographically guided popliteus tendon sheath injection, LAX to the popliteus, and in plane with the transducer. Distal is left, lateral is top. (*B*) Setup for a right knee sonographically guided popliteus tendon sheath injection, SAX to the popliteus and in plane with the transducer. Distal is left, lateral is top. (*C*) Sonographic coronal oblique view of proximal/anterior-to-distal/posterior, popliteus tendon sheath injection, LAX to the tendon and in plane with the transducer. Note that the needle passes through the tendon to the deep side of the tendon sheath. Fibular collateral ligament (FCL) crosses obliquely superficial to the popliteus. (*D*) Sonographic coronal oblique view of distal/anterior-to-proximal/posterior popliteus tendon sheath injection, SAX to the tendon and in plane with the transducer. Note that the SAX approach allows for injection into the deep aspect of the tendon sheath without passing through the tendon.

Needle Approach

- LAX to tendon, in plane: advance proximal/anterior to distal/posterior, entering superficial side of tendon sheath just anterior and deep to FCL (**Fig. 8**C).
- SAX to tendon, in plane: advance distal/anterior to proximal/posterior, to either superficial or deep side of tendon sheath (**Fig. 8**D).

Pearls

- SAX to tendon approach allows injection to deep side of tendon sheath without passing through tendon.
- Given the frequency of asymptomatic popliteus tendinopathy, diagnostic injection can be helpful in evaluation of posterolateral knee pain, although injectate overflow into joint is possible via popliteus hiatus.

PROXIMAL TIBIOFIBULAR JOINT INJECTION
Indications

- Diagnostic and/or therapeutic injection for pain attributed to proximal tibiofibular joint (PTFJ).[1,12]
  - Other diagnostic tests frequently lack specificity to make this diagnosis.
- Avoid injury to the common, superficial, and deep fibular nerves.

Accuracy

One study showed 100% accuracy for USG injection compared with 58% accuracy for LG injection.[12]

Safety

No published complications with this injection.

Clinical Efficacy

No published studies have evaluated or compared the clinical efficacy of USG versus LG injections.

Positioning

- Patient in oblique side-lying position with the knee slightly flexed (**Fig. 9**A).
- Transducer in anatomic transverse oblique plane (medial side pivoted proximally) with its LAX perpendicular to the PTFJ.

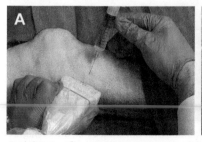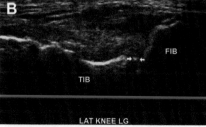

Fig. 9. (*A*) Setup for a right knee sonographically guided PTFJ injection, out of plane with the transducer. Proximal is left, anterior is top. (*B*) Sonographic oblique transverse view of a distal/anterior-to-proximal/posterior injection, out of plane with the transducer, into the PTFJ. Arrows denote needle tip.

Preprocedural scan

- Anchor lateral end of transducer on fibular head with medial end oriented toward inferior patellar pole and rotated to optimize visualization of the PTFJ.[12]
- Anterior superior tibiofibular ligament serves as landmark for the joint space.[12]
- Identify and avoid the common, superficial, and deep fibular nerves.

Needle Approach

Out of plane: distal-to-proximal approach, using a walk-down technique into PTFJ (**Fig. 9**B).

Pearls

Optimal transducer angulation highly variable given interindividual variation in PTFJ orientation.[12]

MEDIAL (TIBIAL) COLLATERAL LIGAMENT BURSA INJECTION
Indications

- Diagnostic and/or therapeutic injection for pain attributed to MCL bursopathy.[13]
- Avoid inadvertent injection into adjacent soft tissues or knee joint.

Accuracy

No published studies have evaluated or compared USG versus LG injections.

Safety

No published complications with this injection.

Clinical Efficacy

No published studies have evaluated or compared the clinical efficacy of USG versus LG injections.

Positioning

- Patient supine with the hip externally rotated and knee slightly flexed (**Fig. 10**A).
- Transducer in anatomic coronal plane over the medial joint line.

Preprocedural Scan

Transducer translated anteriorly and posteriorly to optimally visualize the bursal space lying between the superficial and deep MCL fibers.

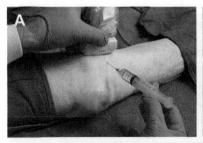 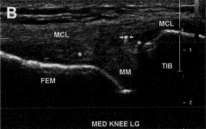

Fig. 10. (A) Setup for a right knee sonographically guided MCL bursa injection, out of plane with the transducer. Proximal is left, medial is top. (B) Sonographic coronal/longitudinal view of an anterior-to-posterior MCL bursa injection, out of plane with the transducer. The needle tip (*arrows*) is visualized deep to the traversing superficial MCL and superficial to the deep MCL (asterisks) and the medial meniscus (MM) in its SAX, between the distal femur and proximal tibia.

Needle Approach

Out of plane: advance anterior to posterior deep to superficial MCL fibers and into bursa (**Fig. 10B**).

Pearls

Initial lidocaine injection can be used to confirm flow within bursal plane.

SEMIMEMBRANOSUS BURSA INJECTION
Indications

- Diagnostic and/or therapeutic injection for pain attributed to SM tendinopathy/bursopathy.[14]
- Identification and avoidance of the saphenous nerve and its branches.

Accuracy

- Onishi and colleagues[14] showed 100% accuracy of USG SM bursa injections.
- No published studies have compared USG with LG injections.

Safety

No published complications with this injection.

Clinical Efficacy

No published studies have evaluated or compared the clinical efficacy of USG versus LG injections.

Positioning

- Patient lateral recumbent with bottom knee partially flexed to optimize imaging of the distal SM tendon (**Fig. 11A**).
- Transducer transverse to SM tendon at level of posteromedial tibial plateau, parallel to the popliteal crease.

Preprocedural Scan

- Trace SM tendon in SAX just proximal to division of anterior and direct arms.
- Identify and avoid saphenous nerve and its branches.

Needle Approach

In plane/Out of plane: advance anterior/proximal to posterior/distal to interval between SM tendon and posteromedial tibia (**Fig. 11B, C**).

Pearls

Placing towel under lateral midfoot internally rotates tibia and relaxes SM, facilitating injectate flow throughout bursa (**Fig. 11D**).

ANTERIOR CRUCIATE LIGAMENT INJECTION
Indications

Direct delivery of medication or regenerative agent into the anterior cruciate ligament (ACL) for therapeutic purposes (eg, partial tear).[15,16]

Accuracy

Smith and colleagues[15] showed 100% accuracy of USG ACL injections. Although fluoroscopically guided (FG) ACL injections are performed in practice, there are no published studies of LG ACL injection accuracy.

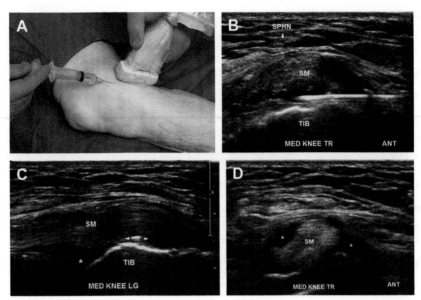

Fig. 11. (*A*) Setup for a right knee sonographically guided SM bursa injection, SAX to the SM tendon, and in plane with the transducer. Proximal is upper left, medial is top. (*B*) Sonographic transverse view of a proximal/anterior-to-distal/posterior injection, in plane with the transducer, and into the SM bursa, which is deep to the SM tendon in its SAX. Note the proximity of the saphenous nerve (SPHN). (*C*) Sonographic longitudinal view of a proximal/anterior-to-distal/posterior injection, out of plane with the transducer, and into the SM bursa (*asterisk*). Needle tip (*arrows*) is deep to the SM tendon, which is in its LAX as it inserts into the tibia. (*D*) Sonographic transverse view of injectate distending the SM bursa (*asterisk*).

Safety

No published complications with this injection.

Clinical Efficacy

Small case series (7 out of 10 patients) showed improvements in pain, function, and ACL MRI appearance after FG bone marrow concentrate injections for ACL sprains and partial tears. No published studies have evaluated the clinical efficacy of USG ACL injections.[16]

Positioning

- Patient supine with the knee flexed to at least 90° and the tibia in slight internal rotation to increase tension on the ACL (**Fig. 12A**).
- Transducer initially placed in anatomic coronal plane over medial joint line near MCL. Final position is in oblique sagittal orientation inferomedial to patella.

Preprocedural Scan

- Beginning in anatomic coronal plane over medial joint line, transducer is translated anteriorly toward patellar tendon.
- As the sagittal plane and patellar tendon are approached, the distal ACL can be identified in oblique orientation ~1 cm deep to anterior tibial cortex.
- ACL will appear hypoechoic because of anisotropy.

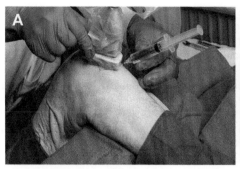
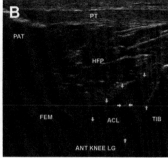

Fig. 12. (*A*) Setup for a right knee sonographically guided ACL injection, LAX to the ligament, and in plane with the transducer. Proximal is left, anterior is top. (*B*) Sonographic sagittal oblique view of an anterior cruciate ligament injection (*yellow arrows* indicate needle tip), in plane with the transducer, with the ACL (*green arrows*) in LAX. Femur, tibia, HFP, patella, and patellar tendon are all visible.

- Proximal end of transducer rotated laterally ~30° (toward inferior pole of patella) to align with orientation of ACL.

Needle Approach

In plane: distal/anterior to proximal/posterior approach, LAX to the ACL, passing medial to patellar tendon, above tibial plateau, and into distal ACL (**Fig. 12**B).

Pearls

- Proximal heel-toe maneuver may improve ACL conspicuity.
- Rotating transducer SAX to ACL/needle tip may facilitate targeting of specific ACL bundle.

SUMMARY

Most structures about the knee region can be accurately targeted for diagnostic or therapeutic injections using USG. The literature consistently reports excellent accuracy using USG to target knee structures, and the use of USG carries many benefits compared with LG injections, such as increased utility with obese patients, diagnostic injection specificity, safety around neurovascular structures, and precise targeting of disorders. However, the clinical efficacy and cost-effectiveness of USG knee procedures have not been well defined and further research in this area is warranted.

REFERENCES

1. Malanga G, Halperin J, Finnoff J, et al. Ultrasound-guided lower limb procedures. Fourth annual hands-on diagnostic and interventional musculoskeletal ultrasound. Rochester (MN): Mayo Clinic/AIUM; 2010.
2. Curtiss HM, Finnoff JT, Peck E, et al. Accuracy of ultrasound-guided and palpation-guided knee injections by an experienced and less-experienced injector using a superolateral approach: a cadaveric study. PM R 2011;3(6):507–15.
3. Park Y, Lee SC, Nam HS, et al. Comparison of sonographically guided intra-articular injections at 3 different sites of the knee. J Ultrasound Med 2011;30(12):1669–76.

4. Bum Park Y, Ah Choi W, Kim YK, et al. Accuracy of blind versus ultrasound-guided suprapatellar bursal injection. J Clin Ultrasound 2012;40(1):20–5.

5. Sibbitt WL Jr, Band PA, Kettwich LG, et al. A randomized controlled trial evaluating the cost-effectiveness of sonographic guidance for intra-articular injection of the osteoarthritic knee. J Clin Rheumatol 2011;17(8):409–15.

6. Tresley J, Jose J. Sonographically guided posteromedial approach for intra-articular knee injections: a safe, accurate, and efficient method. J Ultrasound Med 2015;34(4):721–6.

7. Wisniewski SJ, Murthy N, Smith J. Ultrasound evaluation of Baker cysts: diagnosis and management. PM R 2012;4(7):533–7.

8. Smith MK, Lesniak B, Baraga MG, et al. Treatment of popliteal (Baker) cysts with ultrasound-guided aspiration, fenestration, and injection: long-term follow-up. Sports Health 2015;7(5):409–14.

9. Jelsing EJ, Maida E, Finnoff JT, et al. The source of fluid deep to the iliotibial band: documentation of a potential intra-articular source. PM R 2014;6(2): 134–8 [quiz: 138].

10. Finnoff JT, Nutz DJ, Henning PT, et al. Accuracy of ultrasound-guided versus unguided pes anserinus bursa injections. PM R 2010;2(8):732–9.

11. Smith J, Finnoff JT, Santaella-Sante B, et al. Sonographically guided popliteus tendon sheath injection: techniques and accuracy. J Ultrasound Med 2010; 29(5):775–82.

12. Smith J, Finnoff JT, Levy BA, et al. Sonographically guided proximal tibiofibular joint injection: technique and accuracy. J Ultrasound Med 2010;29(5):783–9.

13. Jose J, Schallert E, Lesniak B. Sonographically guided therapeutic injection for primary medial (tibial) collateral bursitis. J Ultrasound Med 2011;30(2):257–61.

14. Onishi K, Sellon JL, Smith J. Sonographically guided semimembranosus bursa injection: technique and validation. PM R 2016;8(1):51–7.

15. Smith J, Hackel JG, Khan U, et al. Sonographically guided anterior cruciate ligament injection: technique and validation. PM R 2015;7(7):736–45.

16. Centeno CJ, Pitts J, Al-Sayegh H, et al. Anterior cruciate ligament tears treated with percutaneous injection of autologous bone marrow nucleated cells: a case series. J Pain Res 2015;8:437–47.

Ultrasound-Guided Foot and Ankle Procedures

P. Troy Henning, DO

KEYWORDS

• Ankle • Foot • Injection • Ultrasound guidance

KEY POINTS

- Ultrasound-guided injections about the foot and ankle can be used to assist in the alleviation of pain related to disorders of joints, bursae, tendons, and neurologic structures.
- Improved accuracy with ultrasound-guided injections about the foot and ankle allows these procedures to aid in the confirmation of a diagnosis as well as to improve safety, especially when performed adjacent to neurovascular structures.
- Clinicians should be familiar with alternative approaches for various ultrasound-guided procedures about the foot and ankle, because challenging individual patient anatomy or other factors may warrant modification of technique.

TIBIOTALAR (ANKLE) JOINT INJECTION
Regional Anatomy

The tibiotalar joint is a synovial hinge joint formed by the articulation of the tibia and fibula with the underlying talus. The joint recess extends proximally from the inferior tibial margin by a mean of 19.2 mm.[1] An intra-articular extrasynovial fat pad lies within the anterior recess. In addition, the ankle joint communicates with the posterior subtalar joint in 13.9% of cases.[2] From medial to lateral, the tibialis anterior tendon, extensor hallucis longus tendon, dorsalis pedis artery and adjacent deep peroneal nerve, extensor digitorum longus tendon, superficial peroneal nerve, and peroneus tertius tendon overlie the anterior ankle joint.

Patient and Ultrasound Machine Positioning

- Patient: supine on table, injected side closest to provider
- Ultrasound machine: ipsilateral to involved side/provider

Transducer Type

- High-frequency linear-array: small footprint preferred

Conflicts of interest: This author has no financial, professional or personal conflicts to report.
Department of Physical Medicine and Rehabilitation, University of Michigan, 325 East Eisenhower, Ann Arbor, MI 48108, USA
E-mail address: troy.psu@gmail.com

Needle Choice

- Injection only: needle 25 to 30 gauge, 25 to 38 mm
- Aspiration: at least 18-gauge, 38-mm needle

Injectate

Solution of local anesthetic plus corticosteroid (eg, 3 mL of 0.2% ropivacaine and 1 mL of 10 mg/mL triamcinolone).

Approaches

Long axis to joint in plane with transducer

Transducer is aligned in a sagittal plane with the joint overlying the dome of talus (**Fig. 1**). The needle is advanced in an anterior-to-posterior direction deep to the fat pad and superficial to the articular cartilage on the dome of talus, preferably avoiding overlying tendons and neurovascular structures (**Figs. 2–4**).[3]

Short axis to the joint in plane with transducer (the author's preferred approach)

The transducer is aligned in an axial plane with the joint overlying the dome of talus. The needle is advanced in a lateral-to-medial direction deep to the fat pad and superficial to the articular cartilage on the dome of talus, preferably avoiding overlying tendons and neurovascular structures (**Figs. 5–7**).

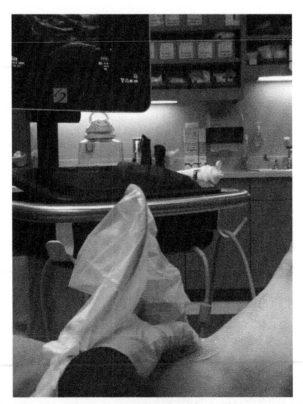

Fig. 1. Position of ultrasound transducer and machine for ankle joint injection in plane with joint. Left, proximal; right, distal.

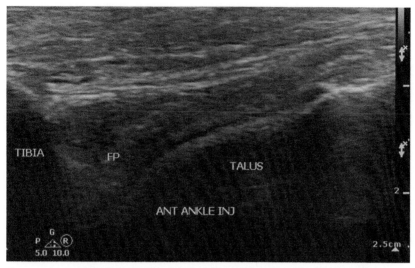

Fig. 2. Anterior ankle joint. Left, proximal; right, distal. Ant, anterior; FP, fat pad.

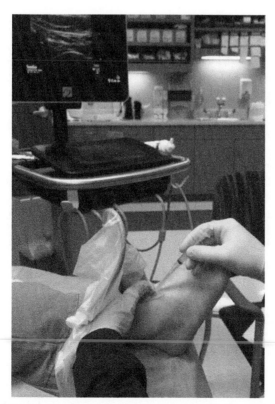

Fig. 3. Ultrasound transducer placement and needle approach for ankle joint injection, in plane with ankle, needle approaching in plane with transducer. Left, proximal; right, distal.

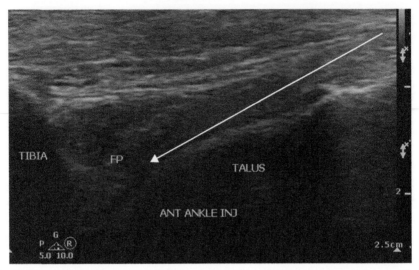

Fig. 4. Sonographically guided injection of the ankle joint, long axis to joint, needle in plane with transducer. Arrow delineates path of needle. Left, proximal; right, distal.

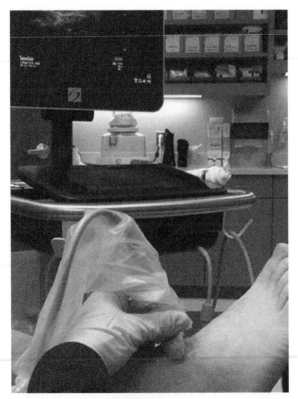

Fig. 5. Transducer position for ankle joint injection, short axis relative to joint. Left, proximal; right, distal.

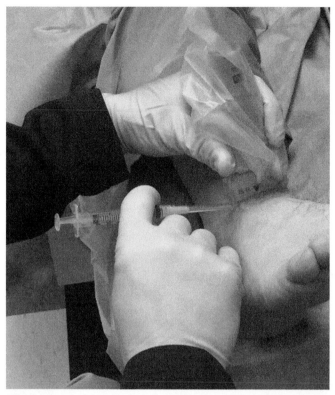

Fig. 6. Ultrasound transducer placement and needle approach for ankle joint injection, short axis to joint, needle in plane with transducer. Left, lateral; right, medial.

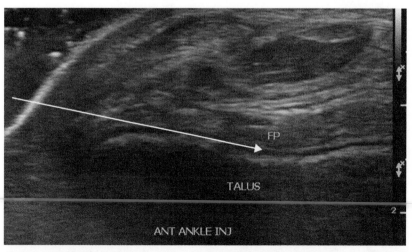

Fig. 7. Sonographically guided injection of ankle joint, short axis to joint, needle in plane with transducer. Arrow delineates path of needle. Note gel standoff window to left of skin to improve placement of the needle. Left, lateral; right, medial.

Long axis to the joint out of plane with transducer (technically more challenging)
The transducer is aligned in a sagittal plane with the joint overlying the dome of talus. Using a walk-down technique from superficial to deep, the needle is advanced in either a lateral-to-medial or an anterior-to-posterior direction deep to the fat pad and superficial to the articular cartilage on the dome of talus, preferably avoiding overlying tendons and neurovascular structures (**Figs. 8** and **9**).

POSTERIOR SUBTALAR JOINT INJECTION
Regional Anatomy

The subtalar joint is a synovial joint between the overlying talus and underlying calcaneus. This joint is divided into 3 facets: anterior, medial, and posterior. Of these, the posterior facet has the largest area and is the focus of this procedure. The flexor hallucis longus (FHL) tendon along with the tibial neurovascular structures overlie the medial aspect of the joint. Laterally, the calcaneofibular ligament and peroneal tendons overlie the joint with the sural nerve traversing just posterior and caudal to the joint. Posteriorly, the Achilles tendon and Kager fat pad are found superficial to the joint.

Patient and Ultrasound Machine Position

Positioning of the patient and ultrasound machine depends on the approach for the injection of this joint, and is discussed further later in this article.

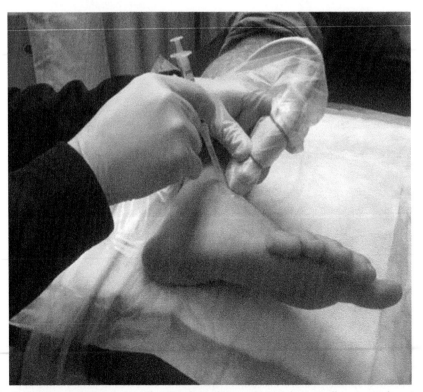

Fig. 8. Ankle joint injection, with transducer long axis to joint, needle approach out of plane with transducer. Left, plantar; right, dorsal.

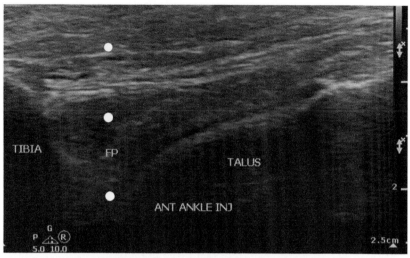

Fig. 9. Sonographically guided injection of ankle joint, long axis to joint, needle path out of plane with transducer. Dots represent path of needle. Each dot signifies a pass of the needle tip below the ultrasound beam. The needle is directed along a steeper trajectory with each pass until the tip is visualized deep to the FP. Left, proximal; right, distal.

Transducer Type

- High-frequency linear-array: short footprint preferable

Needle

- From 25 to 27 gauge, 32 to 51 mm
  - Longer needle (51 mm) likely needed for posterolateral approach

Injectate

- Solution of local anesthetic plus corticosteroid (eg, 1 mL of 0.2% ropivacaine and 1 mL of 10 mg/mL triamcinolone)

Approaches

Posteromedial

The patient position is lateral recumbent, affected side down with the lateral aspect of the ankle resting on a towel or pillow to slightly evert the ankle and open the joint space.[4]

The ultrasound machine is ideally placed posterior to the patient with the provider sitting on the anterior side facing the ultrasound machine and ankle.

The transducer is initially placed over the medial malleolus bridging to the sustentaculum tali. It is then swept posteriorly until the posterior subtalar joint opening is visualized (**Fig. 10**). Immediately overlying the joint, the FHL tendon and tibial neurovascular structures can typically be visualized. The needle is advanced in an anterior-to-posterior direction, out of plane relative to the transducer. A slightly caudal entry position relative to the joint may be needed to avoid the neurovascular structures (**Figs. 11** and **12**).

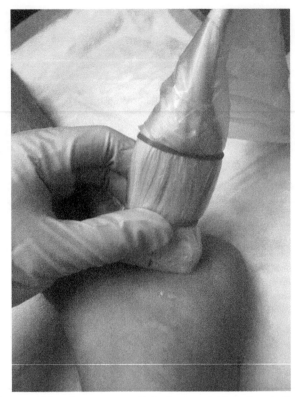

Fig. 10. Transducer position for posteromedial subtalar joint injection. Left, proximal; right, distal.

Anterolateral

The patient position is lateral recumbent, affected side up with the medial side of the ankle resting on a towel or pillow to induce slight inversion of the ankle to open the joint.[4]

The ultrasound machine is ideally placed posterior to the patient with the provider facing the screen and the anterior aspect of the ankle.

The transducer is initially placed overlying the distal fibula and calcaneofibular ligament (**Fig. 13**). Deep to the ligament, the opening of the posterior subtalar joint is easily visualized. The peroneal tendons overlie the ligament with the sural nerve being just caudal and posterior to the joint. The needle is advanced from anterior to posterior, out of plane relative to the transducer (**Figs. 14** and **15**).

Posterolateral

The patient position is prone with the affected ankle dangling off the end of the examination table.[4] Slight passive dorsiflexion of the ankle may help with optimizing access to the joint recess.

The ultrasound machine is ideally located contralateral to the involved ankle with the provider sitting ipsilateral to the involved ankle.

The transducer is placed in the sagittal plane just lateral to the Achilles tendon (**Fig. 16**). The transducer face is angled in a slight medial direction to allow for visualization of the posterior aspects of the tibia, talus, and calcaneus. The needle is

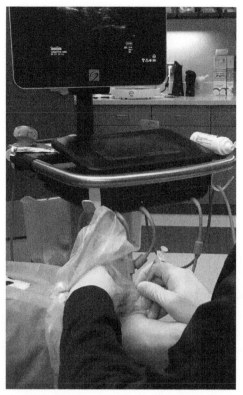

Fig. 11. Posteromedial subtalar joint injection. Transducer short axis to joint, needle approach out of plane with transducer.

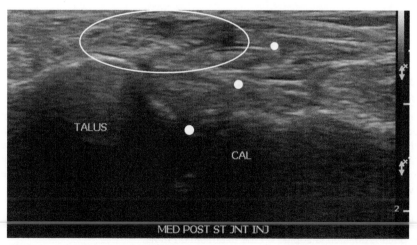

Fig. 12. Posteromedial posterior subtalar joint injection, short axis to joint, needle path out of plane with transducer. Oval encircles the tibial neurovascular structures. Dots represent path of needle. Each dot signifies a pass of the needle tip below the ultrasound beam. The needle is directed along a steeper trajectory with each pass until the tip is visualized within the joint space. Left, superior; right, inferior. CAL, calcaneus.

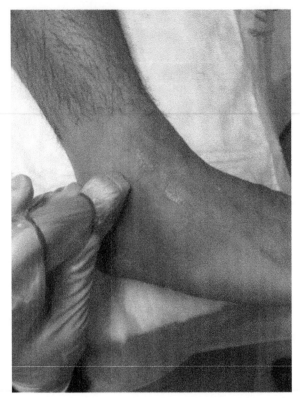

Fig. 13. Transducer position for anterolateral subtalar joint injection. Right, distal and inferior; left, proximal.

inserted in a posterolateral direction, in plane with the transducer (**Fig. 17**). The posterior subtalar joint recess is visualized just deep to the Kager fat pad by visually following the posterior cortex of the calcaneus up to the joint space (**Fig. 18**).

MIDFOOT AND FOREFOOT JOINT INJECTIONS
Regional Anatomy

The midfoot and forefoot joints are synovial joints that are subject to similar disease processes as the hindfoot. Most commonly, patients present with localized pain and swelling related to arthritis or a crystalline disease process. The joints are usually easier to view and access from a dorsal approach. Overlying structures can include the extensor tendons of the toes and branches of the superficial and deep peroneal nerves along with their vascular components.

Patient Position

The patient position is supine on the examination table.

Ultrasound Machine Position

In general, the machine is placed ipsilateral to the involved side with the provider sitting facing the foot with the monitor easily viewed.

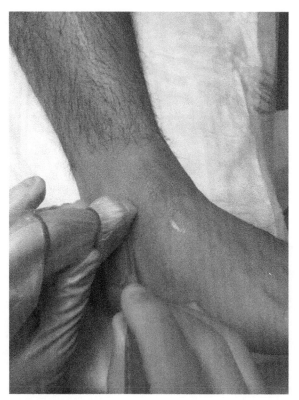

Fig. 14. Injection of anterolateral subtalar joint, transducer short axis to joint, needle out of plane with transducer. Left, proximal; right, distal.

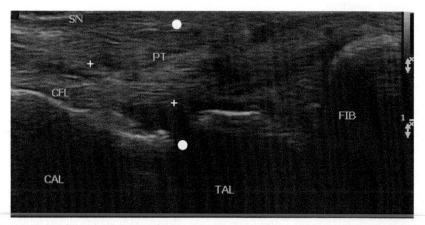

Fig. 15. Anterolateral posterior subtalar joint injection, short axis to joint, needle path out of plane with transducer. Dots represent path of needle. Each dot signifies a pass of the needle tip below the ultrasound beam. The needle is directed along a steeper trajectory with each pass until the tip is visualized within the joint space. The crosses indicate the distance between sural nerve and joint space. Left, inferior; right, superior. CFL, calcaneofibular ligament; FIB, lateral malleolus of fibula; PT, posterior tibial tendon; SN, sural nerve; TAL, talus.

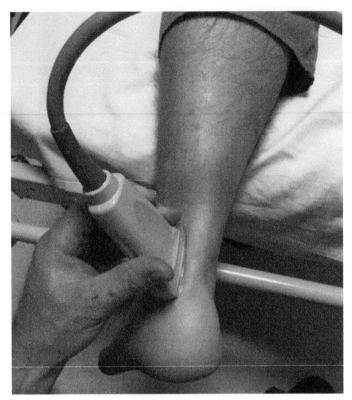

Fig. 16. Transducer position for posterolateral subtalar joint injection. Left, lateral; right, medial.

Transducer Selection

High-frequency linear-array, short-footprint devices are preferred.

Needle

- Injection only: needle 25 to 30-gauge, 25 to 38-mm
- Aspiration: 18-gauge, 38-mm needle

Injectate

Anesthetic with or without corticosteroid; volume may depend on the size of the joint and amount of degenerative changes, where applicable.

Approaches

The joints can be approached from distal to proximal, lateral to medial, or medial to lateral.[5] The best approach depends on the target joint, patient size, and the regional anatomy overlying the joint. Careful preinjection ultrasound scanning allows providers to determine the safest, most efficient window for needle insertion. This author generally uses and recommends an in-plane approach relative to the transducer, but an out-of-plane approach is used if the needle path is limited by overlying structures. Regardless of the approach used, the ultimate goal is to place the needle tip within the joint space, and below the level of the joint capsule (**Figs. 19** and **20**).

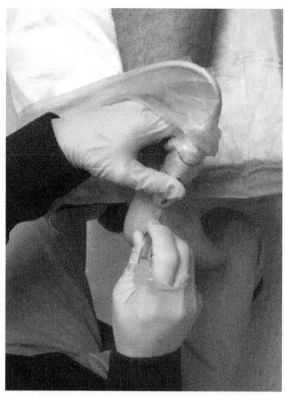

Fig. 17. Posterolateral subtalar joint injection, transducer short axis to joint, needle in plane with transducer. Left, lateral; right, medial.

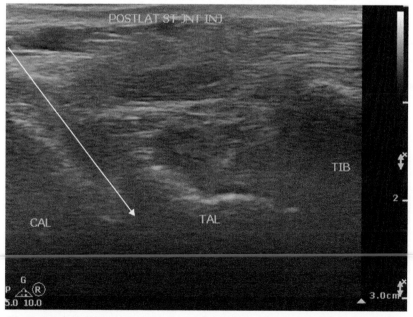

Fig. 18. Posterolateral posterior subtalar joint injection, long axis to joint, needle in plane with transducer. Arrow delineates path of needle. Left, inferior; right, superior. TIB, tibia.

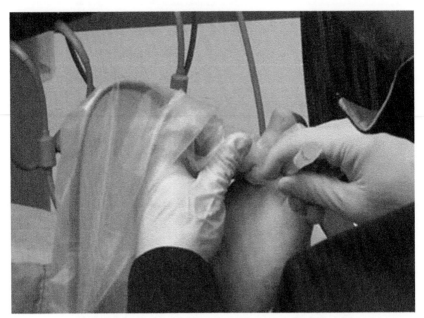

Fig. 19. Metatarsophalangeal joint injection, transducer long axis to joint, needle approaching in plane with transducer. Left, proximal; right, distal.

TENDON SHEATH INJECTIONS
Regional Anatomy

Typical tendon sheath targets include the peroneus longus and brevis; overlap of the FHL and flexor digitorum longus in the foot (master knot of Henry); tibialis anterior; and, in rare cases, the posterior tibial tendon. As a general rule, the author avoids injection of corticosteroid in the posterior tibial tendon sheath because of concerns regarding its propensity to rupture. Although, technically, the plantar fascia does not have a sheath, this structure is typically a target for corticosteroid injections or other related procedures.

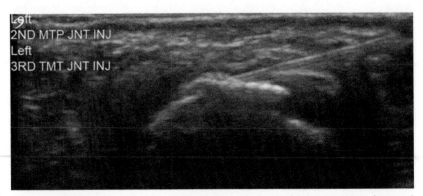

Fig. 20. Sonographically guided second metatarsophalangeal joint injection, long axis to joint, needle in plane with transducer. Left, medial; right, lateral.

When present, a tendon sheath effusion can aid in placement of the needle tip. If no effusion is present, the sheath can gently be filled with careful placement of the needle tip adjacent to the target tendon. Along the lateral foot and ankle, clinicians should account for the sural nerve when approaching the peroneal tendon sheath. Medially, the tibial neurovascular structures need to be identified before the procedure.

Patient Position

Positioning depends on the target; in general, the foot and ankle are placed in a manner that optimizes visualization of the target and allows easier placement of the injectate.

Ultrasound Machine and Provider Position

The ultrasound machine is generally located ipsilateral to the involved side with the provider seated facing the foot and ankle and able to easily visualize the monitor and hands.

Transducer

High-frequency linear-array, short-footprint transducers are preferred.

Needle

A needle of 25 to 30 gauge and 25 to 38 mm is used.

Injectate

Local anesthetic with corticosteroid; volumes may vary by tendon sheath injected and individual patient anatomy.

Approaches

Flexor hallucis longus tendon sheath
Patient position The patient position is prone with a foot hanging over the examination table.

Transducer position Transducer position is in the axial plane to the lower leg and medial to the Achilles tendon. Depth of field of view and focal zones are adjusted to allow visualization of the FHL tendon as it courses past the talus (**Fig. 21**).

Needle approach The needle enters the skin just lateral to the Achilles tendon and is directed through the Kager fat pad into the FHL tendon sheath (**Fig. 22**).

Peroneal tendon sheath
Patient position The patient position is lateral recumbent with the involved side up.

Transducer position The transducer position is axial to the tendons. The tendon sheaths can be injected anywhere along their course, from just proximal to the lateral malleolus to along the region of the foot.

Needle approach The needle can be directed in plane with the transducer in either an anterior or posterior direction depending on the location of the injection. In general, when injecting above the level of the lateral malleolus, it is easier to approach from posterior to anterior (**Figs. 23** and **24**). This direction is in contradistinction to that used when injecting below the level of the malleolus, where an anterior-to-posterior approach is recommended to help avoid the adjacent sural nerve (**Figs. 25** and **26**).

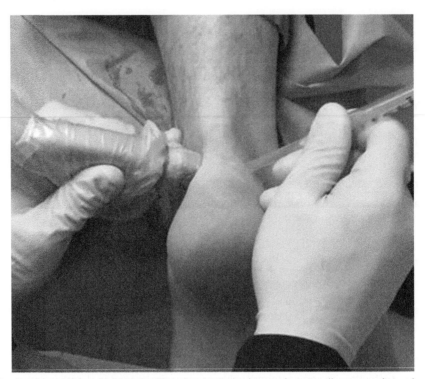

Fig. 21. FHL tendon sheath injection, short axis to the tendon, needle approach in plane with transducer. Left, medial; right, lateral.

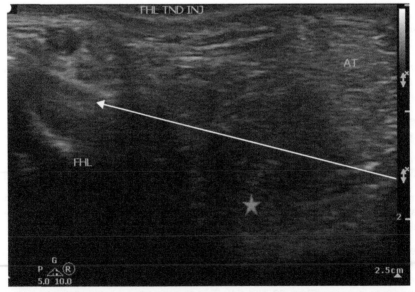

Fig. 22. Sonographically guided flexor hallucis longus tendon sheath injection, short axis to the FHL tendon and Achilles tendon (AT), needle approach in plane with transducer. Arrow delineates path of needle. Star, Kager fat pad. Left, medial; right, lateral.

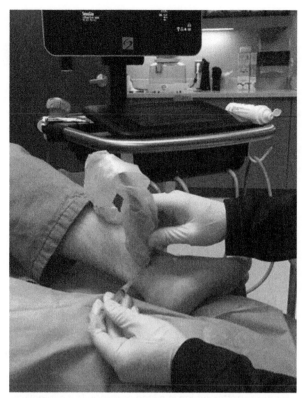

Fig. 23. Peroneal tendon sheath injection proximal to malleolus, short axis to the tendons, needle approach in plane with transducer. Left, proximal; right, distal.

Plantar fascia injection

Patient position The patient position is prone a with foot hanging off the examination table.

Transducer position The transducer can be placed long axis or short axis in reference to the plantar fascia (**Fig. 27**).

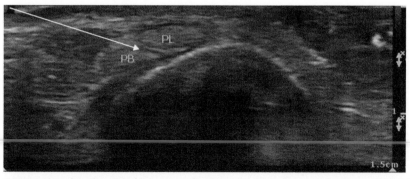

Fig. 24. Sonographically guided injection of peroneal tendon sheath at location proximal to lateral malleolus, short axis to peroneus longus (PL) and peroneus brevis (PB) tendons, needle approach in plane with transducer. Arrow delineates path of needle. Left, posterior; right, anterior.

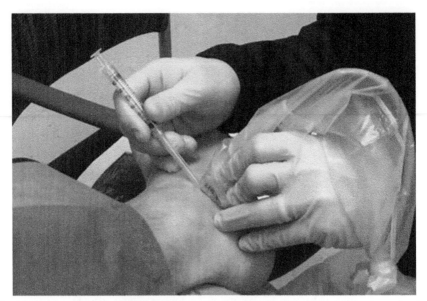

Fig. 25. Peroneal tendon sheath injection distal to lateral malleolus, short axis to the tendons, needle approach in plane with transducer. Left, proximal; right, distal.

Needle approach The approach depends on the desired outcome. It can be advanced in or out of plane with the transducer, from a medial/lateral or proximal/distal direction (**Fig. 28**). The needle and solution can be delivered superficial to, within, or deep to the plantar fascia.[6] Delivering an injection deep to the plantar fascia can also allow for treatment of Baxter neuropathy, which is a less common but clinically important cause of chronic heel pain.[7]

BURSA INJECTION
Regional Anatomy

The retrocalcaneal and retro-Achilles bursae are targets for injection about the hindfoot. On occasion, an adventitial bursa about the foot and ankle may be present, usually along the first metatarsophalangeal joint or plantar to the metatarsal heads.[8]

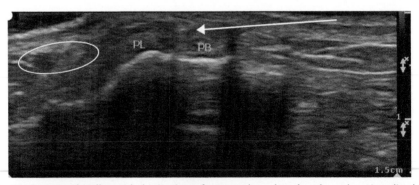

Fig. 26. Sonographically guided injection of peroneal tendon sheaths at location distal to lateral malleolus. Imaged short axis to PL and PB tendons, needle approach in plane with transducer. Arrow delineates path of needle. Oval encircles sural nerve and vein. Left, inferior and posterior; right, anterior and superior.

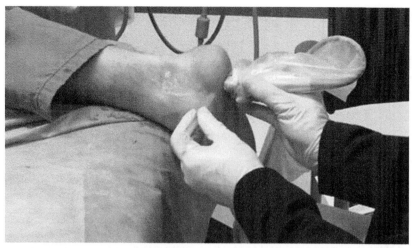

Fig. 27. Plantar fascia injection, short axis to plantar fascia origin, needle approach in plane with transducer. Left, proximal; right, distal.

Patient Position

The patient position is prone or supine depending on the location of the target bursa.

Ultrasound Machine/Provider Location

Ipsilateral to the involved bursa, the provider faces the foot, with the ability to visualize the monitor and hands.

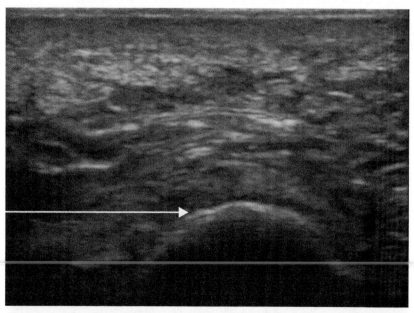

Fig. 28. Sonographically guided plantar fascia injection. Arrow denotes needle path. Needle tip placed just deep to plantar fascia just distal to medial calcaneal tubercle. Left, medial; right, lateral.

Transducer

A high-frequency linear-array transducer is used.

Needle

- Injection only: a needle of 25 to 30 gauge, 25 to 38 mm.
- Aspiration: 18-gauge, 38-mm needle.

Approach

In or out of plane relative to the transducer. The needle can be advanced from either a medial or lateral direction into the desired bursa (**Figs. 29** and **30**).

INTERDIGITAL NEUROMA OF FOOT
Regional Anatomy

An interdigital neuroma of the foot involves the common plantar digital nerves, which are derived from the medial and lateral plantar nerves. Most frequently, neuromas are found at the third intermetatarsal space; a neuroma in this specific interdigital space is known as a Morton neuroma. This location is related to several factors: the common plantar nerve here forms from contributions of both the medial and lateral plantar nerves, the third metatarsal space is narrower than the other metatarsal spaces, and the third and fourth metatarsals tend to be more mobile relative to the other metatarsals.[9] Corticosteroid injections for symptomatic interdigital neuromas can potentially provide relief of pain for up to 3 months.[10]

Patient and Ultrasound Machine Position

The patient is supine with the machine ipsilateral to the involved side, and the provider is facing the foot with the ability to visualize the monitor and hands.

Transducer

A high-frequency linear-array transducer is used.

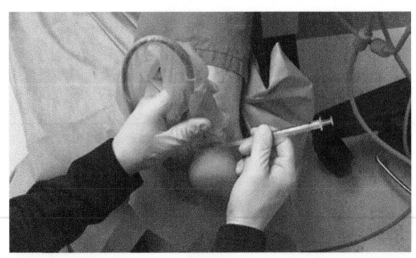

Fig. 29. Retro-Achilles or retrocalcaneal bursa injection, short axis to bursa, needle approach in plane with transducer. Right, lateral; left, medial.

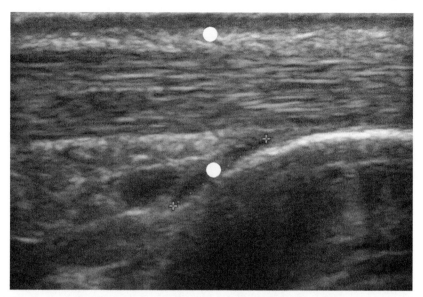

Fig. 30. Sonographically guided retro-Achilles or retrocalcaneal bursa injection with out-of-plane approach depicted. The dots represent walk-down technique with needle to target bursa; in this example, the retrocalcaneal bursa is highlighted by crosses. Left, proximal; right, distal.

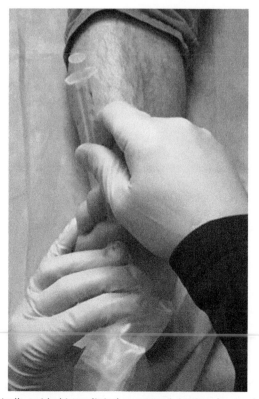

Fig. 31. Sonographically guided interdigital neuroma injection, long axis to neuroma, needle approach in plane with transducer. Left, lateral; right, medial.

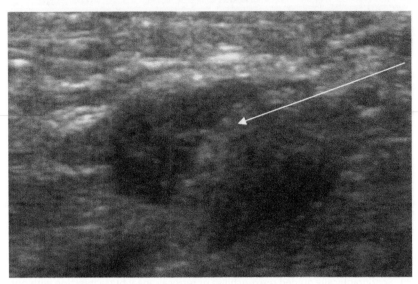

Fig. 32. Sonographically guided interdigital neuroma injection, long axis to neuroma, needle approach in plane with transducer. Arrow delineates path of needle. Left, proximal; right, distal.

Needle

A needle of 25 to 30 gauge and 25 to 38 mm is used.

Approach

Distal to proximal in plane with the transducer, the needle enters between the toes along the plantar side of the interdigital space (**Figs. 31** and **32**). The transducer can be placed on the dorsal or plantar aspect of the foot.

SUMMARY

Injections about the foot and ankle are commonly performed in musculoskeletal practice. Using sonographic guidance can improve the accuracy and potentially increase the safety of these procedures. Although this article is not exhaustive in describing ultrasound-guided injection techniques about the foot and ankle, it can serve as a good foundation from which to develop approaches when targeting other structures.

REFERENCES

1. Lee PTH. The proximal extent of the ankle capsule and safety for the insertion of percutaneous fine wires. J Bone Joint Surg Br 2005;87(5):668.
2. Carmont MR, Tomlinson JE, Blundell C, et al. Variability of joint communications in the foot and ankle demonstrated by contrast-enhanced diagnostic injections. Foot Ankle Int 2009;30(5):439.
3. Wisniewski SJ, Smith J, Patterson DG, et al. Ultrasound-guided versus nonguided tibiotalar joint and sinus tarsi injections: a cadaveric study. PM R 2010;2(4):277.
4. Henning T, Finnoff JT, Smith J. Sonographically guided posterior subtalar joint injections: anatomic study and validation of 3 approaches. PM R 2009;1(10):925.

5. Sahler CS, Spinner DA, Kirschner JS. Ultrasound-guided first metatarsophalangeal joint injections: description of an in-plane, gel standoff technique in a cadaveric study. Foot Ankle Spec 2013;6(4):303.
6. Kayhan A, Gökay NS, Alpaslan R. Sonographically guided corticosteroid injection for treatment of plantar fasciosis. J Ultrasound Med 2011;30(4):509–15.
7. Maida E, Presley JC, Murthy N, et al. Sonographically guided deep plantar fascia injections: where does the injectate go? J Ultrasound Med 2013;32(8):1451.
8. Van Hul E, Vanhoenacker F, Van Dyck P, et al. Pseudotumoural soft tissue lesions of the foot and ankle: a pictorial review. Insights Imaging 2011;2(4):439.
9. Bianchi S, Martinoli C. Ultrasound of the musculoskeletal system. Springer; 2007. p. 1–974.
10. Thomson CE, Beggs I, Martin DJ, et al. Methylprednisolone injections for the treatment of Morton neuroma. J Bone Joint Surg Am 2013;95(9):790.

Ultrasound-Guided Spinal Procedures for Pain
A Review

Mark-Friedrich B. Hurdle, MD[a,b,*]

KEYWORDS

- Epidural • Facet • Interventional spine • Interventional pain • Pain management
- Sonography • Spine injections • Ultrasonography

KEY POINTS

- Ultrasound (US) has become a more common imaging modality for spinal interventions.
- US has some advantages and disadvantages compared with fluoroscopy and other imaging modalities.
- Most typical spinal pain procedures described under fluoroscopy have also been described with US guidance.
- Although there are multiple studies demonstrating the accuracy of US-guided spine procedures using cadaveric dissections as well as comparing their accuracy to procedures with CT or fluoroscopic guidance, there are no large studies comparing the safety or efficacy of US-guided spinal interventions to CT or fluoroscopic guidance.
- Some spinal interventions where the spinal vascular supply may be at risk may still benefit from fluoroscopic or CT-confirmed contrast-controlled verification.

INTRODUCTION

The aging population presents musculoskeletal clinicians with an increasing incidence of degenerative changes of the spine and associated pain. Although interventional spine procedures have been in use for decades, common imaging modalities have relied on ionizing radiation for guidance. US has more recently become used to image axial structures and guide procedures in this region.

Like other imaging modalities, US has certain advantages and disadvantages. US imaging is ideal for visualizing soft tissues, bony surfaces, and needle manipulation

Disclosures: The author has no disclosures.
[a] Department of Physical Medicine and Rehabilitation, Mayo Clinic, 4500 San Pablo Road, Jacksonville, FL 32224, USA; [b] Department of Pain Medicine, Mayo Clinic, 4500 San Pablo Road, Jacksonville, FL 32224, USA
* Department of Physical Medicine and Rehabilitation, Mayo Clinic, 4500 San Pablo Road, Jacksonville, FL 32224.
E-mail address: hurdle.markfriedrich@mayo.edu

in real time. Significant nerves and blood vessels can readily be visualized by a well-trained sonographer. Unfortunately, the deeper the tissue, the more challenging sonographic visualization becomes. In addition, bone completely obstructs US visualization of deeper structures in the path of sound waves. As such, clinicians should consider US one of several options for image guidance for spine procedures.

ULTRASOUND-GUIDED CERVICAL SPINE PROCEDURES
Anatomy

The cervical spine is composed of 7 vertebral levels with the atlanto-occipital (C0-C1) and atlantoaxial (C1-C2) having unique anatomic features. This article's focus is on the middle and lower cervical joints. Potential pain generators at each level include the vertebral body, facets, nerve roots, and disks. Under US guidance, the cervical facets and medial branches are relatively accessible in most patients.[1] At the C2-C3 level, the facet may refer pain to the third occipital nerve (TON), which may also be blocked.[2]

Indications

The cervical facets can be prominent pain generators in patients with both occipital and posterior neck pain. This pain can be related to osteoarthritic and whiplash injuries.[3] Facetogenic pain may be present despite normal CT, bone scan, or MRI findings. In whiplash-induced neck pain, medial branch blocks of the cervical facets are often needed to confirm the correct pain generator. Common interventions for facetogenic pain in the cervical spine include facet injections, medial branch blocks, and radiofrequency ablation of the medial branches.[4]

Technique

Ultrasound-guided technique for identification of the correct cervical level for cervical facet injections

The patient is placed in the lateral decubitus position with the side of interest facing upward. Typically, a high-frequency (>10 MHz) linear-array transducer is used in the axial plane to scan the lateral neck starting caudally (**Fig. 1**). The posterior tubercle of the segmental foramen can be well visualized. The C7 foramen can be localized because there is no prominent anterior tubercle (**Fig. 2**). The other cervical foramina have prominent anterior tubercles. At the C6 foramen, the C5-C6 facet is visualized. The needle then is advanced in-plane using an anterior-to-posterior approach. A posterior approach using a low-frequency (<10 MHz) curvilinear-array transducer in the prone position has also been described.[5]

Ultrasound-guided technique for cervical medial branch blocks and third occipital nerve blocks

For a TON block, the patient is placed in the lateral decubitus position and the transducer is placed in the coronal plane with the cephalic end of the transducer on the mastoid process. Next the transducer is moved 5 mm to 8 mm posteriorly until the articular pillar of C2 is well visualized (**Fig. 3**). The transducer is then translated caudally until the C2-C3 articulation along with the TON is visualized (**Fig. 4**).[2] To visualize the more caudal medial branches, the transducer can be translated caudally while maintaining a coronal view. The hyperechoic peaks with a cleft are articular processes and joints, whereas the hyperechoic valleys are where the medial branches lie. In an out-of-plane approach, a short 25-gauge needle can be advanced from anterior to posterior, targeting the deepest point in the near-contiguous hyperechoic bony

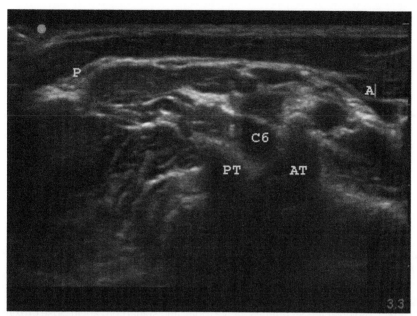

Fig. 1. Axial plane US image of the neck at the C6 level. Note that the vertebral artery is obscured by bone at this level. A, anterior; AT, anterior tubercle; C6, C6 nerve root; P, posterior; PT, posterior tubercle.

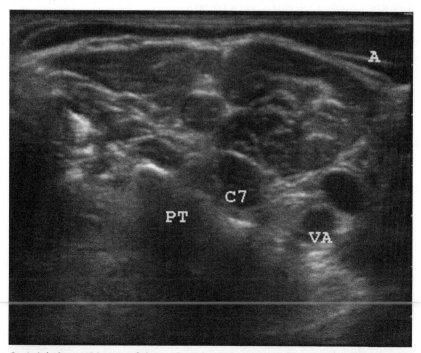

Fig. 2. Axial plane US image of the neck at the C7 level. Note that the vertebral artery is not obscured by bone at this level. A, anterior; C7, C7 nerve root; PT, posterior tubercle; VA, vertebral artery.

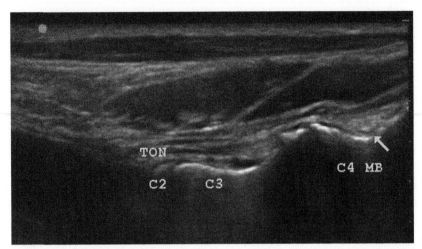

Fig. 3. Coronal plane US image of the TON. The nerve sits on the joint between C2 and C3. (*Arrow*) C4 medial branch (MB).

ridge.[6] Only 0.3 mL of a local anesthetic is needed under direct observation. The vertebral artery, radicular feeder arteries, nerve roots, and spinal cord are in close proximity to these structures, and clinicians should take appropriate precautions to carefully avoid them.

ULTRASOUND-GUIDED THORACIC PROCEDURES
Anatomy

The thoracic spine is composed of 12 vertebral levels. Thoracic back pain is not as common as lumbar or cervical pain; however, it is present in approximately 15% of

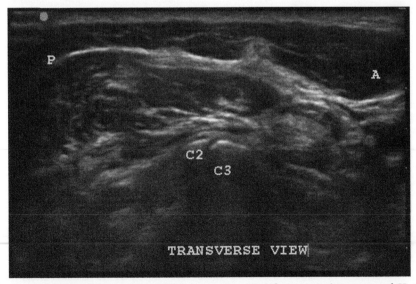

Fig. 4. Axial plane US image of the TON. A, anterior; C2, inferior articular process of C2; C3, SAP of C3; P, posterior.

adults. This pain can be chronic and severe.[7] Common pain generators include the disks, facets, and nerve roots. Additional sources of pain, however, include the costovertebral and costotransverse joints. With US imaging alone, the disks and costovertebral joints are not commonly injected due to poor visualization. US-guided facet and costotransverse joint injections, however, have been described.[8,9]

Indications

Thoracic joint injections are usually performed to treat inflamed, painful, arthritic facets and costotransverse joints. If conservative options fail, CT, bone scan, or MRI can be used to help localize the pain generator. Because of the close proximity of the disks and facet, costotransverse, and costovertebral joints to each other at each segment, it is frequently difficult to isolate the pain generator using physical examination alone.

Technique

Ultrasound-guided technique for thoracic facet injections
A key to completing successful thoracic facet injections is isolating the correct level. Caudal-to-cranial scanning is used to locate the 12th rib on the affected side. In the sagittal plane, the 12th rib is followed medially until the costotransverse joint is visualized. When translating the transducer slightly more medially, the hyperechoic lamina of the 12th vertebra becomes visible. The transducer is then moved in a cephalic direction while counting laminar levels until the level of choice has been located. At this point, while still in the sagittal plane, the transducer is tilted medially so the US beam is aiming slightly lateral (**Fig. 5**). The sawtooth pattern of the facets then comes into view. At this point, the skin is marked to delineate the transducer location and needle entry site caudally. The needle is subsequently advanced in a caudal-to-cephalic fashion into the joint.

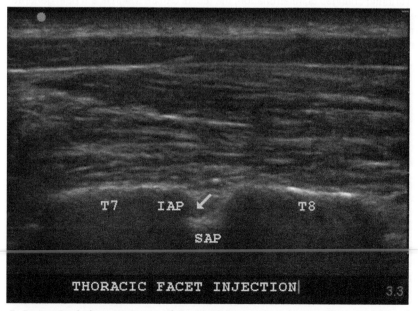

Fig. 5. Parasagittal plane US image of the T7-T8 facet. IAP, inferior articular process of T7; SAP, SAP of T8; *arrow*, joint space of the facet joint.

Ultrasound-guided technique for costotransverse joint injections

The patient is placed in the prone position. As described previously with the thoracic facets, caudal-to-cranial scanning in the sagittal plane is used to identify the 12th rib on the side of interest. The ribs can then be counted until the level of interest has been reached. The transducer is then rotated directly over until the rib and transducer are parallel. The rib is then followed medially until the costotransverse joint is visualized (**Fig. 6**). The skin is marked to verify the position of the transducer. After the skin is prepped in the usual sterile fashion, a 22-gauge spinal needle is advanced in-plane in a lateral-to-medial approach into the joint.

ULTRASOUND-GUIDED LUMBAR SPINE PROCEDURES

Lumbar pain and radicular leg pain are leading reasons people seek treatment with their primary care provider.[10,11] Typical treatment options include physical therapy, oral analgesic/anti-inflammatory medications, and injection therapies. Recently, image-guided interventions have become common among pain specialists.[12] Over the past decade, more evidence is building that US is a viable imaging modality for lumbar spinal procedures.[13,14]

Anatomy

The lumbar spine is composed of 5 vertebral levels separated by disks anteriorly. These disks can become a source of pain, or they can compress adjacent nerve roots causing neuropathic pain. Posteriorly, the lumbar facet joints are composed of the inferior articular process of the more cephalic level and the superior articular process (SAP) of the more caudal level. These facet joints are diarthrodial, containing hyaline cartilage and a synovial lining.

Indications

With arthritic changes or inflammation, the facets can be a significant pain generator.[15] Skeletal imaging, such as MRI, plain x-ray films, or CT scan, is needed to confirm the number of lumbar vertebrae prior to any US-guided lumbar intervention, because anatomic anomalies can affect procedural performance and safety.

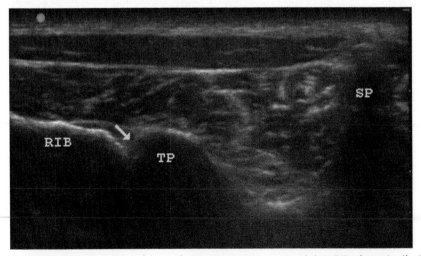

Fig. 6. Axial plane US image of (*arrow*) costotransverse process joint. RIB, thoracic rib; SP, spinous process.

Technique

Ultrasound-guided technique for identification of the correct lumbar level for lumbar facet injections and medial branch blocks

The patient is placed in the prone position with either 1 or 2 pillows under the lower abdomen to flex the lumbar spine for optimal visualization. Usually, a low-frequency (<10-MHz) curvilinear-array transducer is used to obtain sufficient sonographic penetration. The transducer is placed over the midline in a sagittal plane at the lumbosacral junction to visualize the lumbar spinous processes and the crest of S1. The lumbar spinous processes can be counted and labeled on the skin. The transducer can then be translated laterally, maintaining a strict sagittal view until a contiguous sawtooth pattern is observed (**Fig. 7**). This long-axis view of the spine shows a series of more superficial rounded hyperechoic facets in series (**Fig. 8**). Just lateral to the facets and parallel to the spine in a slightly deeper plane, the medial transverse processes (TPs) come into view (**Fig. 9**).

After identifying and marking lumbar levels in the longitudinal view, the transducer can be rotated 90° to view the spine in an axial plane (**Fig. 10**). At the level of the sacral crest, the S1 foramina and posterior superior iliac crest can be visualized. Maintaining an axial plane and translating the transducer cephalically, the interlaminar space and dura come into view medially. Laterally, the L5-S1 facet and sacral ala become visible. With the cephalic scan, the L4-L5 facets come into view. By translating the transducer laterally, the TP can be seen in the axial plane.

Technique for ultrasound-guided lumbar facet injections

The patient is placed in the prone position and the lumbar spine is scanned in the sagittal and axial planes (as outlined previously). Special attention is given to correctly mark the lumbar levels and the lumbosacral junction. The facet of interest can be identified by scanning in between the spinous processes of the target level in the axial plane and scanning slightly laterally to visualize the facet on the affected side. The transducer position is marked and the skin is then prepped and draped in the usual sterile fashion. After the skin is anesthetized, a 22-gauge spinal needle is advanced from lateral-to-medial into the joint.[16] The more cephalic lumbar facet joints typically have a more sagittal orientation than the more caudal joints.

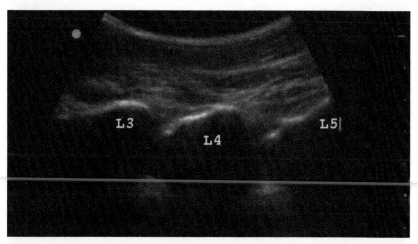

Fig. 7. Parasagittal view of the lumbar spine where the lamina is seen in a sawtooth pattern. L3, L4, L5, the lamina of the respective lumbar vertebral levels.

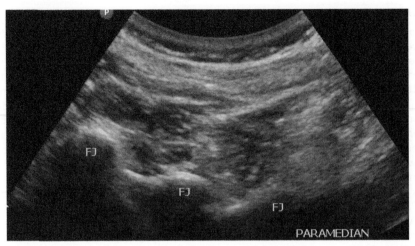

Fig. 8. Parasagittal plane US image of lumbar facet joints, lateral to lamina. FJ, lumbar facet joints in succession.

Technique for ultrasound-guided lumbar medial branch blocks

The patient is placed in the prone position and the lumbar spine is scanned in the sagittal and axial planes (as outlined previously). Once the spinous processes are correctly marked, the transducer is placed over the level of interest in the axial plane and is translated laterally until the SAP and the TPs are visualized. The transducer position is marked and the skin is the prepped and draped in the usual sterile fashion. The skin is properly anesthetized prior to advancing a 22-gauge spinal needle medially, targeting the angle between the SAP and TP. Once a bony endpoint has been established, the transducer is rotated 90° (parasagittal) to ensure the needle tip has a cephalic position on the TP.[14,17]

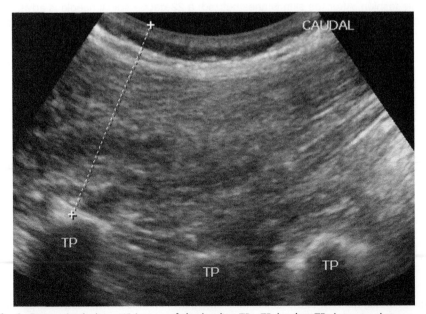

Fig. 9. Parasagittal plane US image of the lumbar TPs. TP, lumbar TPs in succession.

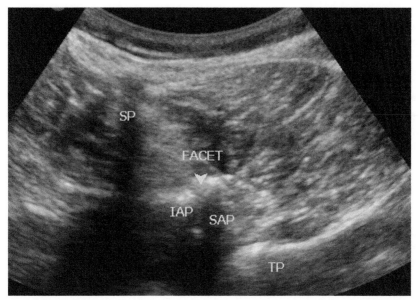

Fig. 10. Axial plane US image of the lumbar facets. IAP, inferior articular process; SP, spinous process; *arrowhead*, lumbar facet.

ULTRASOUND-GUIDED SACROILIAC JOINT INJECTIONS
Anatomy

The sacroiliac joint (SIJ) links the spine to the pelvis. Typically, the more caudal portion of the joint has true synovium, whereas the more proximal portion may contain only fibrocartilage.[18] The posterior SIJ is innervated by the dorsal S2-S4 nerve roots, whereas the anterior joint is innervated by the L2-S2 nerve roots.[19]

Indications

Typically, patients present with pain in the area of the rejoin of the SIJ. Provocative maneuvers and imaging studies do not provide highly reliable diagnostic information with regard to pain generation. Currently, a diagnostic injection of the SIJ can provide clinicians with more reliable data.[20]

US-guided SIJ blocks were described by Pekkafahli and colleagues[21] with CT confirmation. The investigators described a significant learning curve with a 60% success rate in the initial 30 injections and a 93.5% success rate in the subsequent 30 injections. A feasibility study using CT confirmation published in 2008 showed a higher success rate at the caudal pole SIJ injections in cadavers compared with a more cephalic approach.[22] In the same study using live patients (10 injections), the success rate was 100%.

Technique

The patient is placed the prone position and the area of interest is exposed. The posterior superior iliac spine (PSIS) can be palpated as the most prominent bony landmark slightly lateral to midline and just caudal to the lumbosacral junction. Once the transducer has been placed over the PSIS in the axial plane, the SIJ can be observed by slowly scanning caudally as the step-off between the sacrum and ilium becomes less pronounced. Eventually, the ilium is no longer visible once the transducer is over the sciatic notch. At this point, the transducer's direction is changed, rescanning in the cephalic direction until the ilium is visualized. This scanning technique helps confirm the caudal pole SIJ injection (**Fig. 11**). Next, a 22-gauge spinal needle is advanced from the medial side of the transducer using an in-plane approach into the SIJ.

ULTRASOUND-GUIDED CAUDAL EPIDURAL INJECTIONS
Anatomy

Typically, the sacral hiatus can be located around the level of S4 and S5 along the midline of the posterior sacrum. The sacral cornua create the lateral borders of the hiatus whereas the posterior sacrum creates the floor. Distally, the hiatus is covered by the sacrococcygeal ligament. The epidural space extends all the way to the sacral hiatus whereas typically the dura only extends to the S2 level. The anterior component of the sacral epidural space tends to be the most vascular.[23]

Indications

Typically, caudal epidural injections are considered when patients have had multilevel posterior spinal fusion with poor epidural access. Patients also may be suffering from chronic and diffuse lumbosacral, leg, or pelvic pain.

Technique

US-guided caudal epidural injections have been described by Yoon and colleagues.[24] The patient is placed in the prone position. Typically, the sacral cornua can be palpated just lateral to midline along the distal sacrum. A high-frequency (>10-MHz) linear-array transducer is placed directly over the cornua so they can be visualized as 2 prominent hyperechoic osseous structures connected via a thinner hyperechoic sacrococcygeal ligament (**Fig. 12**). Next, the transducer is pivoted 90° while maintaining a midline view between the cornua (**Fig. 13**). A 22-gauge spinal needle is then advanced in-plane between the dorsal sacral plate and the anterior sacrum into the sacral canal. Unfortunately, there is no highly reliable method using US to verify the needle is accurately positioned in the epidural space and not in a vascular structure. This US-guided technique may be used when contrast is contraindicated or fluoroscopy alone proves challenging.

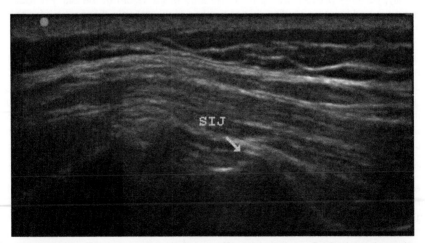

Fig. 11. Axial plane US image of the inferior pole of the SIJ (*arrow*). The lateral sacral crest is medial to the joint, whereas the iliac crest is lateral to the joint. Left, medial; right, lateral.

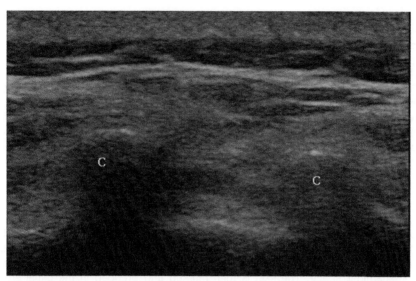

Fig. 12. Axial plane US image of the sacral cornua. The sacral cornua in short axis are depicted by the hyperechoic line above both letters, C. The hyperechoic line between the cornua represents the sacrococcygeal ligament just superficial to the sacral hiatus.

ULTRASOUND-GUIDED INTERLAMINAR EPIDURAL INJECTIONS
Anatomy

At the level of the thoracic spine, there are 12 interlaminar spaces posteriorly between T1 and L1. The spinous processes of the thoracic spine slope caudally covering a significant portion of the posterior interlaminar opening. In addition, the ligamentum flavum may be absent at the midline in the upper thoracic spine.[25] At the lumbosacral

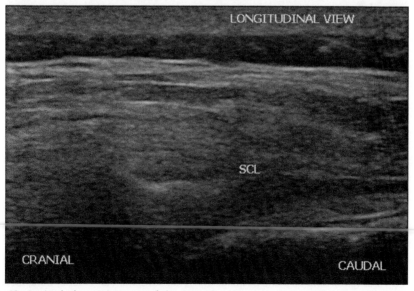

Fig. 13. Sagittal plane US image of the posterior sacrum in the position used for a caudal epidural injection. SCL, sacrococcygeal ligament.

level, there are 5 posterior openings between L1 and the sacrum. The largest opening is typically at the L5-S1 level. With age, the ligamentum flavum frequently becomes thicker.[26]

Indications

Epidural injections have been used in both the acute and chronic setting to control pain.[27,28] Typically, there is a radicular component to the pain in the chronic setting. Advanced imaging can show discrete neural compromise or inflammation that correlates with the location of the symptoms. In the lumbar spine, a provocative physical examination maneuver, such as a straight leg raise, can help confirm the diagnosis of radiculopathy.

Technique

Lumbar and thoracic epidural injections have been described by Grau and colleagues[29] in the literature.[30] The patient is placed in the prone position with the thoracolumbar spine flexed. For the thoracic spine, the ribs are counted to verify the correct level (as discussed previously). A view of the facets is obtained in the parasagittal plane. The transducer is then tilted so that the US beam is directed medially into the interlaminar space. The skin is then marked and prepped in the usual sterile fashion. After the administration of local anesthetic, a Tuohy spinal needle is advanced from the caudal to cephalic position. Once the needle is advanced past the lamina medially, a loss-of-resistance technique is used. A third hand is required to assist with either holding the transducer or advancing the needle.

For a lumbar epidural injection under US, a similar approach is used.[5] A view of the correct lumbar level is obtained (as outlined previously). Once a view of the facets is obtained in the parasagittal plane, an oblique angle is obtained so that the US beam is aimed medially (**Fig. 14**). The skin is then marked and prepped in a sterile

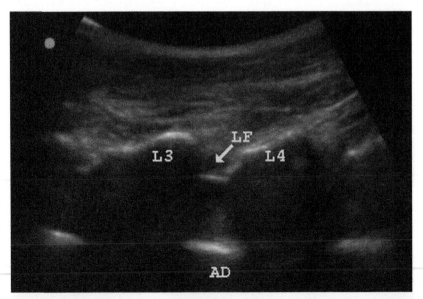

Fig. 14. Parasagittal oblique plane US image of the lumbar spine. AD, anterior dura; L3, lamina of L3; L4, lamina of L4; LF (*arrow*), ligamentum flavum; hyperechoic line deep to ligamentum flavum, posterior dura.

fashion. The skin at the needle entry site is anesthetized. A spinal needle is then advanced from caudal to cephalic directly under the transducer until the needle is imbedded into the denser tissue of the ligamentum flavum. At this point, a loss-of-resistance technique is used with an assistant.

SUMMARY

US has become increasingly common as an imaging modality for spinal interventions. It has advantages and disadvantages versus CT and fluoroscopic guidance and should be considered an option among the interventional spine clinician's repertoire. Large studies comparing the safety and efficacy of US-guided spinal interventions versus CT and fluoroscopy are needed to further define the role of these procedures.

REFERENCES

1. Siegenthaler A, Schliessbach J, Curatolo M, et al. Ultrasound anatomy of the nerves supplying the cervical zygapophyseal joints: an exploratory study. Reg Anesth Pain Med 2011;36(6):606–10.
2. Eichenberger U, Greher M, Kapral S, et al. Sonographic visualization and ultrasound-guided block of the third occipital nerve: prospective for a new method to diagnose C2-C3 zygapophysial joint pain. Anesthesiology 2006; 104(2):303–8.
3. Lord SM, Barnsley L, Wallis BJ, et al. Chronic cervical zygapophysial joint pain after whiplash. A placebo-controlled prevalence study. Spine (Phila Pa 1976) 1996;21(15):1737–44 [discussion: 1744–5].
4. Lord SM, Barnsley L, Wallis BJ, et al. Percutaneous radio-frequency neurotomy for chronic cervical zygapophyseal-joint pain. N Engl J Med 1996;335(23): 1721–6.
5. Narouze S, Peng PW. Ultrasound-guided interventional procedures in pain medicine: a review of anatomy, sonoanatomy, and procedures. Part II: axial structures. Reg Anesth Pain Med 2010;35(4):386–96.
6. Siegenthaler A, Eichenberger U, Curatolo M. A shortened radiofrequency denervation method for cervical zygapophysial joint pain based on ultrasound localization of the nerves. Pain Med 2011;12(12):1703–9.
7. Linton SJ, Hellsing AL, Halldén K. A population-based study of spinal pain among 35-45-year-old individuals. Prevalence, sick leave, and health care use. Spine (Phila Pa 1976) 1998;23(13):1457–63.
8. Stulc SM, Hurdle MF, Pingree MJ, et al. Ultrasound-guided thoracic facet injections: description of a technique. J Ultrasound Med 2011;30(3):357–62.
9. Deimel GW, Hurdle MF, Murthy N, et al. Sonographically guided costotransverse joint injections: a computed tomographically controlled cadaveric feasibility study. J Ultrasound Med 2013;32(12):2083–9.
10. Bogduk N. On the definitions and physiology of back pain, referred pain, and radicular pain. Pain 2009;147(1–3):17–9.
11. Moore AE, Jeffery R, Gray A, et al. An anatomical ultrasound study of the long posterior sacro-iliac ligament. Clin Anat 2010;23(8):971–7.
12. Carrino JA, Morrison WB, Parker L, et al. Spinal injection procedures: volume, provider distribution, and reimbursement in the U.S. medicare population from 1993 to 1999. Radiology 2002;225(3):723–9.
13. Galiano K, Obwegeser AA, Bodner G, et al. Ultrasound guidance for facet joint injections in the lumbar spine: a computed tomography-controlled feasibility study. Anesth Analg 2005;101(2):579–83.

14. Greher M, Kirchmair L, Enna B, et al. Ultrasound-guided lumbar facet nerve block: accuracy of a new technique confirmed by computed tomography. Anesthesiology 2004;101(5):1195–200.
15. Schwarzer AC, Wang SC, Bogduk N, et al. Prevalence and clinical features of lumbar zygapophysial joint pain: a study in an Australian population with chronic low back pain. Ann Rheum Dis 1995;54(2):100–6.
16. Galiano K, Obwegeser AA, Bodner G, et al. Real-time sonographic imaging for periradicular injections in the lumbar spine: a sonographic anatomic study of a new technique. J Ultrasound Med 2005;24(1):33–8.
17. Shim JK, Moon JC, Yoon KB, et al. Ultrasound-guided lumbar medial-branch block: a clinical study with fluoroscopy control. Reg Anesth Pain Med 2006; 31(5):451–4.
18. Forst SL, Wheeler MT, Fortin JD, et al. The sacroiliac joint: anatomy, physiology and clinical significance. Pain Physician 2006;9(1):61–7.
19. Grob D, Panjabi M, Dvorak J, et al. The unstable spine–an "in vitro" and "in vivo" study" on better understanding of clinical instability. Orthopade 1994;23(4):291–8 [in German].
20. Foley BS, Buschbacher RM. Sacroiliac joint pain: anatomy, biomechanics, diagnosis, and treatment. Am J Phys Med Rehabil 2006;85(12):997–1006.
21. Pekkafahli MZ, Kiralp MZ, Başekim CC, et al. Sacroiliac joint injections performed with sonographic guidance. J Ultrasound Med 2003;22(6):553–9.
22. Klauser A, De Zordo T, Feuchtner G, et al. Feasibility of ultrasound-guided sacroiliac joint injection considering sonoanatomic landmarks at two different levels in cadavers and patients. Arthritis Rheum 2008;59(11):1618–24.
23. Senoglu N, Senoglu M, Oksuz H, et al. Landmarks of the sacral hiatus for caudal epidural block: an anatomical study. Br J Anaesth 2005;95(5):692–5.
24. Yoon JS, Sim KH, Kim SJ, et al. The feasibility of color Doppler ultrasonography for caudal epidural steroid injection. Pain 2005;118(1–2):210–4.
25. Lirk P, Kolbitsch C, Putz G, et al. Cervical and high thoracic ligamentum flavum frequently fails to fuse in the midline. Anesthesiology 2003;99(6):1387–90.
26. Capogna G, Celleno D, Simonetti C, et al. Anatomy of the lumbar epidural region using magnetic resonance imaging: a study of dimensions and a comparison of two postures. Int J Obstet Anesth 1997;6(2):97–100.
27. Benyamin RM, Wang VC, Vallejo R, et al. A systematic evaluation of thoracic interlaminar epidural injections. Pain Physician 2012;15(4):E497–514.
28. Armon C, Argoff CE, Samuels J, et al. Subcommittee of the American Academy of Neurology. Assessment: use of epidural steroid injections to treat radicular lumbosacral pain: report of the Therapeutics and Technology Assessment Subcommittee of the American Academy of Neurology. Neurology 2007;68(10): 723–9.
29. Grau T, Leipold RW, Conradi R, et al. Efficacy of ultrasound imaging in obstetric epidural anesthesia. J Clin Anesth 2002;14(3):169–75.
30. Grau T, Leipold RW, Delorme S, et al. Ultrasound imaging of the thoracic epidural space. Reg Anesth Pain Med 2002;27(2):200–6.

Ultrasound-Guided Peripheral Nerve Procedures

Jeffrey A. Strakowski, MD[a,b,c],*

KEYWORDS

- Injection • Intervention • Neurological • Neuroma • Neuropathy • Perineural
- Sonography • Ultrasound

KEY POINTS

- Detailed preprocedural scanning should always be performed before an ultrasound-guided peripheral nerve procedure to determine the ideal approach.
- Ultrasound image optimization is necessary for reliably identifying peripheral nerves and appropriately performing procedures.
- Having all necessary equipment and planning done in advance will facilitate an effective and safe ultrasound-guided peripheral nerve procedure.

INTRODUCTION

Ultrasound guidance allows real-time visualization of the needle in peripheral nerve procedures with improved accuracy and safety. The visualization of the vulnerable target of the peripheral nerve as well as the surrounding anatomy can provide valuable information for both diagnostic purposes and procedure enhancement. Detailed knowledge of the anatomy and appropriate prescanning and equipment preparation can facilitate effective use of ultrasound for peripheral nerve procedures.

Success with peripheral nerve procedures requires knowledge of nerve structure and anatomy, technical skills, and unique challenges associated with peripheral nerves. A thorough knowledge of anatomy, including the peripheral nerve course, function, and surrounding tissue is needed.

Appropriate use of depth, frequency, focal zones, and gray-scale mapping will provide the clearest view of the target region around the peripheral nerve. The depth should be set so the target area takes up the largest portion of the screen. The image

Disclosures: The author has no commercial or financial conflicts of interest.
[a] Department of Physical Medicine and Rehabilitation, The Ohio State University, 480 Medical Center Drive, Columbus, OH 43210, USA; [b] Department of Physical Medicine and Rehabilitation, Riverside Methodist Hospital, 3555 Olentangy River Road, Columbus, OH 43214, USA; [c] The McConnell Spine, Sport, and Joint Center, 3773 Olentangy River Road, Columbus, OH 43214, USA
* 3773 Olentangy River Road, Columbus, OH 43214.
E-mail address: jstrak@aol.com

should be centered to allow adequate visualization of the approach of the needle to the target. Generally, the highest frequency available that still provides adequate penetration to the tissue desired will create the clearest image of the peripheral nerve.[1] The focal zone should be placed at the desired target for the clearest image (**Fig. 1**). The gray-scale mapping is chosen to provide the greatest contrast between the nerve and surrounding tissue. Most peripheral nerve injections are performed with a short-axis view of the nerve and an in-plane view of the needle. This allows the best view of the outline of the nerve and visualization of the approach of the needle. It some situations, it is advantageous to rotate between short-axis and long-axis views of the nerve to establish both vantage points.

The patient should be positioned between the clinician and the ultrasound screen to allow easy visualization of both the needle at the target site and the ultrasound image. The necessary equipment for the injection should be reviewed before the procedure and placed easily within reach. Detailed preprocedural scanning should be performed before the procedure to plan the approach and investigate the surrounding anatomy, including potential anatomic variants.[2]

Peripheral nerves provide unique challenges as an injection target, including borders that can be somewhat indistinct relative to surrounding tissue. Nerves also are relatively mobile and have the potential to move from the initial target site with tissue movement as well as infiltrating injectate. Nerves are also vulnerable targets with considerable potential for injury. Some investigators argue that intraneural injections are relatively safe if the needle does not penetrate the fascicles.[3-5] Despite this, caution is recommended for all injections because of limits of resolution and variability of the pattern of fascicular architecture in some nerves.[6] Creating a halo around the nerve with injectate can increase the conspicuity of nerve borders (**Fig. 2**).[7] Use of blunt needles can also help facilitate safe injections very close to the peripheral nerve borders.

GENERAL PROCEDURAL CONSIDERATIONS

A detailed discussion of all peripheral nerve procedures is beyond the scope of this article. The more commonly performed procedures are discussed. There are often

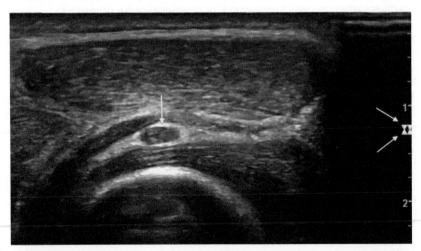

Fig. 1. Sonogram demonstrating a short-axis view of an abnormally enlarged deep branch of the radial nerve (*single arrow*) at the level of the supinator. The focal zone (*double arrows*) is set at the appropriate level for optimization of the image.

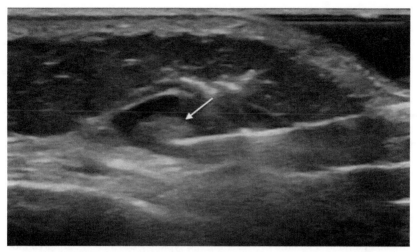

Fig. 2. Sonogram demonstrating the increased conspicuity of a short-axis view of the small saphenous nerve (*arrow*), created by the hypoechoic halo of the injectate. The hyperechoic needle tip is seen just posterior to the nerve.

multiple approaches to performing peripheral nerve injections.[2] The following represent the author's preferred techniques. In all of the following injections, a short-axis view of the nerve and in-plane view of the needle are preferred.

A high-frequency (>10 MHz) linear-array transducer is best for visualization of superficial structures and should be used for most peripheral nerve injections (**Fig. 3**). Peripheral nerve injections always should be performed with sterile technique,

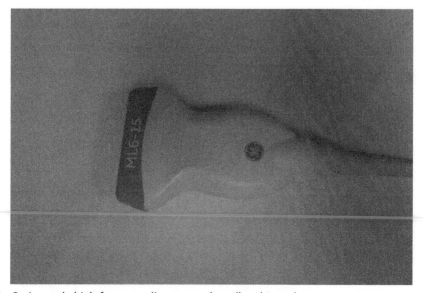

Fig. 3. A sample high-frequency linear-array broadband transducer.

including use of appropriate sterilizing agents for the skin. Alcohol-based chlorhexi-dine for this purpose is preferred over povidone-iodine by many institutions. Use of sterile probe covers can alleviate the need to sterilize the transducer surface (**Fig. 4**). This is generally preferred because it allows free movement of the transducer in the field for optimization of tissue and needle conspicuity.[8] Transducer covers were not used for most of the images in this article for picture clarity.

The transducer always should be maintained in as close to an orthogonal position relative the needle as possible. This will provide the highest conspicuity of the needle. With an in-plane approach, ensure that the needle remains in parallel underneath the transducer. Approach at an oblique angle will result in visibility of only a portion of the needle. The needle should not be advanced if the tip is not visible.[9] The needle direction of many peripheral nerve injections is relatively superficial. Use of an oblique gel stand-off can assist with establishing proper needle trajectory before entry through the skin. This is accomplished by using a large amount of sterile gel on the needle entry side of the transducer.

The injectate used for each procedure is based on the desired intervention. Local anesthetics alone in a volume of 1 to 4 mL are typically used for most nerve blocks. Injectable corticosteroids are often used in conjunction with the anesthetic if the goal is longer relief, particularly in the context of entrapment neuropathies. The flow of the injectate should always be initiated slowly and watched carefully to ensure proper location because of the potential vulnerability of the target. The nerve is often more conspicuous once the initial injectate is placed near the target. Larger volumes of injectate are used for hydrodissection. This can consist of 5 to 15 mL of a combination of normal saline and local anesthetic. Some also use dextrose solution. The literature regarding hydrodissection techniques and whether they provide significant benefit over standard perineural injections is sparse at this time, and further studies are needed to provide better insight into the appropriate indications and methods for this technique.[10–12]

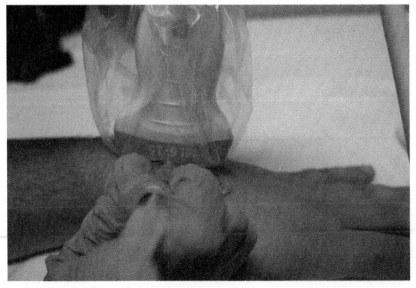

Fig. 4. An example of a sterile transducer cover.

Suprascapular Nerve at the Suprascapular Notch

Indications
Suprascapular nerve injections are most often used to treat intractable shoulder pain. Acutely this often is for postoperative shoulder pain. In the context of chronic shoulder pain, the injections can be used in a context of a diagnostic trial or with longer-acting agents, including anesthetic agents with steroids, toxic agents such as phenol, and radiofrequency ablations. Most injections of the suprascapular nerve are performed at the suprascapular notch. Some investigators advocate a supraclavicular approach.[13] Aspiration of compressive posterior labral cysts are also performed in the area of the spinoglenoid foramen (**Fig. 5**).[14–17]

Anatomy
The suprascapular nerve arises from the C5 and C6 roots and departs the brachial plexus near the location of the convergence of those roots as they form the superior trunk. The nerve travels deep to the trapezius toward the posterior shoulder along the border of the scapula. It becomes visible on ultrasound as it traverses through the suprascapular notch deep to the superior transverse scapular ligament.[18] It is accompanied by the suprascapular artery and vein. It then gives branches to the supraspinatus in the supraspinatus fossa and continues around the lateral border of the spine of the scapula into the infraspinatus fossa. From there it gives branches to the infraspinatus.[19] The suprascapular nerve provides motor innervation to the supraspinatus and infraspinatus as well as sensory innervation to the acromioclavicular and glenohumeral joints.

Scanning
The suprascapular nerve can be visualized with the suprascapular artery and vein at the suprascapular notch and also at the spinoglenoid foramen (**Fig. 6**).[20] The transducer is placed in the plane of the spine of the scapula. Internal and external rotation of the shoulder as well as use of Doppler imaging may help distinguish the suprascapular artery and vein. The hypoechoic suprascapular vein will enlarge and collapse with internal and external rotation.[21] Effort should be made to identify the superior transverse ligament at the suprascapular notch; however, some investigators have

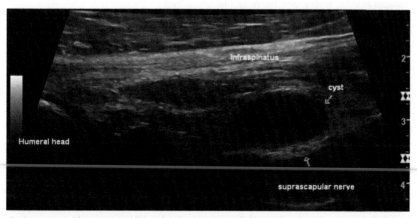

Fig. 5. Sonogram demonstrating a short-axis view of the suprascapular nerve adjacent to a posterior labral cyst at the spinoglenoid fossa. A cyst of this nature can cause neuropathy by compression of the nerve.

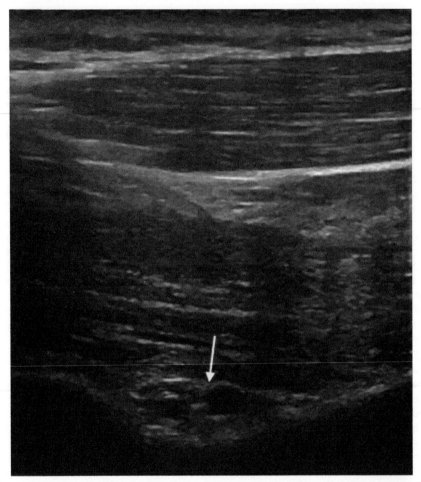

Fig. 6. Sonogram demonstrating a view of the suprascapular notch (*arrow*) where the suprascapular vein, artery, and nerve can be visualized.

suggested that this may be difficult to distinguish sonographically from the fascia of the supraspinatus muscle.[22]

Procedure

a. Needle: 22 gauge, 64 to 89 mm (**Figs. 7** and **8**).[23,24]
b. Patient position:
   i. Seated with the hand on the contralateral shoulder; or
   ii. Prone with the arm hanging off the edge of the table.
c. Transducer position: Parallel to the spine of the scapula over the suprascapular notch.
d. Needle approach: Medial-to-lateral or lateral-to-medial are both effective.
e. Target: Near the suprascapular nerve at the suprascapular notch. The needle should be directed deep to the superior transverse scapular ligament.
f. Avoid: Intravascular injection of the suprascapular artery and vein.
g. Tip: There is often temporary resistance when passing through the superior transverse scapular ligament.

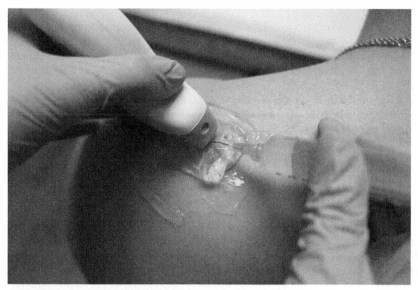

Fig. 7. Arrangement for an injection near the suprascapular nerve at the suprascapular notch.

Deep Branch of the Radial Nerve at the Supinator

Indications

Entrapment of the deep branch of the radial nerve at the supinator is also known as radial tunnel syndrome.[25] It is a controversial source of forearm pain and is considered a possible pain generator in recalcitrant lateral epicondylalgia.[26–28] Measurable neurologic deficit from this location is rarely reported in the absence of trauma or mass. The literature is currently sparse respecting the efficacy of this injection.

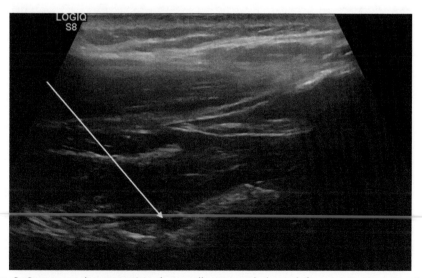

Fig. 8. Sonogram demonstrating the needle approach (*arrow*) for an injection near the suprascapular nerve at the suprascapular notch.

Anatomy

The radial nerve bifurcates into the deep branch of the radial nerve and the superficial radial sensory nerve near the level of the radiocapitellar joint. The deep branch of the radial nerve enters the radial tunnel through the Arcade of Frohse (supinator arch), which is the fibrous entrance to the space between the superficial and deep layers of the supinator (**Fig. 9**).[29,30] The nerve becomes the posterior interosseus nerve once it exits the supinator and lies on the posterior interosseus membrane.[31] It innervates the extensor digitorum, extensor digiti minimi, extensor carpi ulnaris, abductor pollicis longus, extensor pollicis longus, extensor pollicis brevis, and extensor indicis. Significant injury to this nerve can result in weakness of digit extension and radial deviation of the wrist with extension.[32] The actual entrapment site in this area is controversial. Many propose that the nerve is typically entrapped as it enters the Arcade of Frohse.[33] Others support entrapment in or at the exit point of the radial tunnel.[34–36]

Scanning

The deep branch of the radial nerve can be identified as it bifurcates from the superficial sensory branch near the elbow joint. It is followed in short-axis toward its entrance to the supinator. The recurrent radial artery and its accompanying veins (Leash of Henry) can be identified before the entrance of the nerve through the Arcade of Frohse.[37] The nerve should then be followed through the exit from the supinator. It should be assessed in both short-axis and long-axis for both focal and diffuse enlargement along its course. Comparison with the presumably unaffected contralateral side should always be done when enlargement is suspected and the precise location of the procedure is being determined (**Fig. 10**).[38]

Procedure

a. Needle: 25 gauge to 27 gauge, 51 to 89 mm (**Figs. 11** and **12**).[2,39]
b. Patient position: Supine or seated with the forearm resting on the table, the elbow slightly flexed, and the thumb pointed upward.

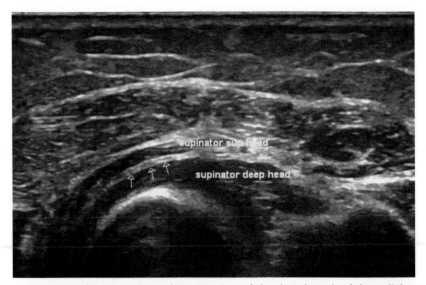

Fig. 9. Sonogram demonstrating a short-axis view of the deep branch of the radial nerve (*arrows*) in the radial tunnel between the deep and superficial heads of the supinator.

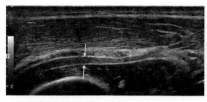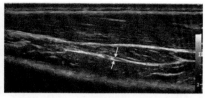

Fig. 10. Sonograms demonstrating long-axis views of the deep branch of the radial nerve (*arrows*) at the level of the supinator in the abnormally enlarged side (*left image*) and normal comparison (*right image*), illustrating the dramatic difference in size.

c. Transducer position: Short-axis for injection. Both short-axis and long-axis often used for hydrodissection.
d. Needle approach: Medial-to-lateral for single injection. Use of medial-to-lateral and also distal-to-proximal for hydrodissection.
e. Target: The deep branch of the radial nerve near an identified focal flattening and proximal swelling. Often between the superficial and deep heads of the supinator.
f. Avoid: Intraneural injection and injury to the recurrent radial artery.

Median Nerve at the Pronator Teres

Indications
Entrapment of the median nerve at the level of the pronator teres is also known as "pronator tunnel syndrome." It is a rare source of median neuropathy and should be considered when there is neurologic deficit involving the median-innervated forearm muscles or pain in the median nerve distribution that is not attributed to median neuropathy at the carpal tunnel. It is reported to present in the absence of neurologic deficit as a vague ache in the forearm that is worsened by repetitive motion.[40]

Because the pronator teres is not a typical entrapment site, such as the much more common carpal tunnel, detailed use of history, physical examination, and when

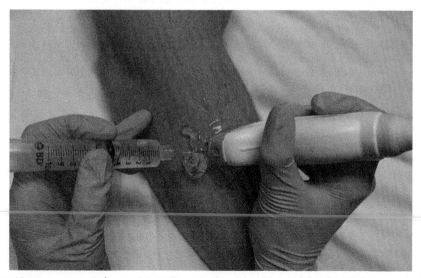

Fig. 11. Arrangement for an injection near the deep branch of the radial nerve at the supinator.

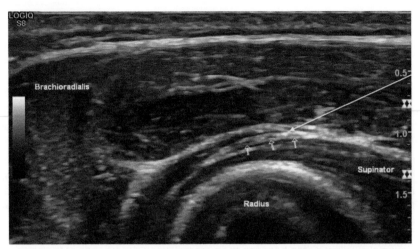

Fig. 12. Sonogram demonstrating the needle approach (*long arrow*) for an injection near the deep branch of the radial nerve (*short arrows*) in short-axis at the supinator.

appropriate, electrodiagnosis and diagnostic imaging should be used to confirm focal neuropathy in this location.[41]

Anatomy

The median nerve is supplied by the cervical roots of C6 to T1. The median nerve traverses the elbow medial to the nearby brachial artery. It passes beneath the lacertus fibrosus and the radial head of the pronator teres, and then between the radial and ulnar heads of the pronator teres.[42] In most individuals, the ulnar artery emerges as a bifurcation from the brachial artery and traverses posterior to the median nerve at the level of the pronator tunnel. The innervations for the flexor carpi radialis, palmaris longus, and flexor digitorum superficialis emerge near the level of the pronator teres.[43] The anterior interosseus nerve typically emerges from the main trunk of the median nerve just after exiting the pronator teres. The main trunk of the median nerve continues distally to innervate the abductor pollicis brevis, opponens pollicis, superficial head of the flexor pollicis brevis, and the first and second lumbricals. It additionally provides cutaneous sensation to the palm and palmar aspect of the thumb, index, and long fingers, as well as the radial side of the ring finger.

Scanning

The nerve should be followed in short-axis view from above the antecubital fossa through the heads of the of the pronator teres (**Fig. 13**). The nerve also should be assessed in long-axis (**Fig. 14**). A heel-toe maneuver with the transducer can reduce anisotropic artifact in the long-axis image.[44] The nearby brachial artery and its ulnar artery branch should be identified for avoidance during the injection.

Procedure

a. Needle: 25 to 27 gauge, 38 to 64 mm (**Figs. 15** and **16**).[2,45]
b. Patient position: Seated or supine with the forearm resting on the table in supinated position and the elbow relatively extended.
c. Transducer position: Short-axis for injection. Both short-axis and long-axis often used for hydrodissection.

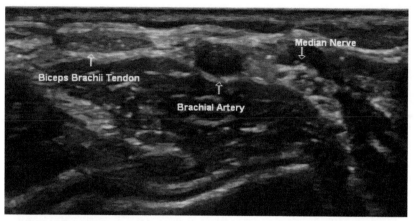

Fig. 13. Sonogram of a short-axis view of the median nerve just proximal to its entrance into the pronator tunnel.

d. Needle approach: Medial-to-lateral for single injection. Use of medial-to-lateral and also distal-to-proximal for hydrodissection.
e. Target: The median nerve near an identified focal flattening and proximal swelling. Often between the radial and ulnar heads of the pronator teres.
f. Avoid: An intraneural injection of the median nerve. Also identify and avoid the more lateral brachial artery proximally and the bifurcation and path of the ulnar artery at the more distal path of the median nerve. Identification of the anterior interosseus nerve and artery is needed when injecting at the more distal aspect of the pronator tunnel.

Median Nerve at the Carpal Tunnel

Indications
Entrapment of the median nerve at the carpal tunnel is the most common and well-defined neuropathy in the human body and is known as carpal tunnel syndrome. Clinical, electrophysiologic, and imaging techniques facilitate diagnosis of this condition with a high degree of accuracy.[46–49] Use of localized steroid injections have been

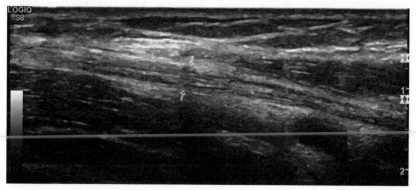

Fig. 14. Sonogram demonstrating a long-axis view of the median nerve (*arrows*) at the level of its entrance to the pronator tunnel.

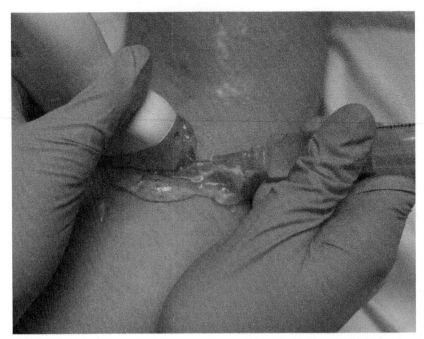

Fig. 15. Arrangement for an injection near the median nerve at the level of the pronator tunnel.

shown to be an effective intervention for providing symptomatic relief.[50] There has been growing interest in the use of hydrodissection for this condition.

Anatomy

The carpal tunnel space is bordered by the carpal bones on the radial, ulnar, and dorsal sides. The volar aspect is covered by the transverse carpal ligament. The carpal tunnel also contains the tendon of the flexor pollicis longus, the 4 flexor digitorum

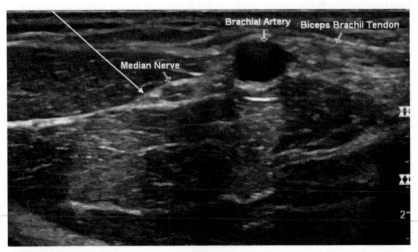

Fig. 16. Sonogram demonstrating the needle approach (*long arrow*) for an injection near the median nerve in short-axis at the level of the pronator tunnel.

superficialis tendons, and the 4 flexor digitorum profundus tendons. The ulnar tunnel lies to the ulnar side of the wrist and contains the ulnar artery and nerve (**Fig. 17**).[51] The median nerve enters the carpal tunnel space at the carpal tunnel inlet. This is identified on imaging with the bony landmarks of the scaphoid, lunate, and pisiform (**Fig. 18**).[52] This is frequently the site of abnormal enlargement of the median nerve.[53] In neuropathy at the carpal tunnel, the nerve is typically flattened at the carpal tunnel outlet where the transverse carpal ligament is generally thicker (**Fig. 19**).[54] The carpal tunnel outlet is identified by the bony landmarks of the trapezium on the radial side and hamate on the ulnar side.

Scanning
The median nerve should be followed from the forearm through the carpal tunnel space before the injection. The carpal tunnel inlet and outlet should be identified and the relative position of the median nerve to the ulnar artery and nerve should be assessed.[55] The median nerve should be examined for focal flattening and enlargement.[56,57] The nerve should be investigated for the relatively common variant of an early bifurcation creating a bifid appearance.[58,59] A persistent median artery also can be seen either with or without an early bifurcation (**Fig. 20**).[60] Identification of these relatively common anatomic variants can prevent inadvertent neurovascular injury.[61]

Procedure
a. Needle: 25 gauge, 25 to 38 mm (**Figs. 21** and **22**).[62,63]
b. Patient position: Seated or supine with the forearm in supination and the wrist in slight dorsiflexion.
c. Transducer position: Short-axis to the median nerve and carpal tunnel space.
d. Needle approach: Medial-to-lateral.
e. Target: The area around the median nerve, including both dorsal and palmar sides.
f. Avoid: An intraneural injection of the median nerve or the ulnar artery or nerve.

Lateral Cutaneous Nerve of the Thigh

Indications
Neuropathy of the lateral cutaneous nerve of the thigh can result in pain and sensory disturbance affecting a cutaneous distribution in the anterolateral thigh.[64] This

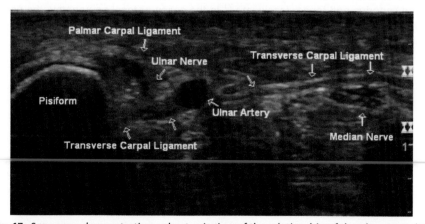

Fig. 17. Sonogram demonstrating a short-axis view of the relationship of the ulnar tunnel to the carpal tunnel.

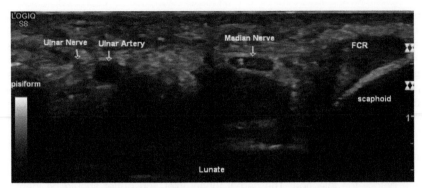

Fig. 18. Sonogram demonstrating a short-axis view of the carpal tunnel inlet.

condition is known as meralgia paresthetica and is typically a result of entrapment of the nerve at the inguinal ligament.[65] Other sources of injury include trauma, stretch, localized compression, or ischemia.

Anatomy
The lateral cutaneous nerve of the thigh is a pure sensory nerve that is derived from the lumbar roots of L2 and L3. It travels along the lateral border of the psoas and exits the pelvis under the inguinal ligament just medial to the anterior superior iliac spine (ASIS) (**Fig. 23**). It then passes through fascia between the sartorius and tensor fascia lata and branches into a cutaneous distribution of a large portion of the anterolateral thigh.[66] It should be noted that there is some individual variability in its location and its relationship to the inguinal ligament.[67,68]

Scanning
The lateral cutaneous nerve of the thigh is a smaller nerve that can be challenging to identify when not enlarged. It can be most easily recognized by sweeping the transducer along the nerve's course while in short-axis over its expected anatomic location.[69] The bony landmark of the ASIS can be seen just lateral to the nerve and the inguinal ligament typically superior to the nerve.[70] The transducer should be moved distally to identify the nerve in a subcutaneous position between the fascial planes of the sartorius and tensor fascia lata.[71] In the cases of focal neuropathy, the nerve is often markedly enlarged, dramatically increasing the conspicuity (**Fig. 24**).

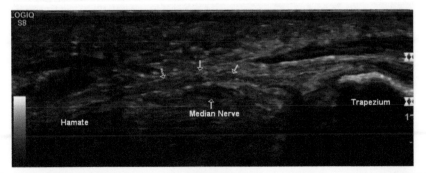

Fig. 19. Sonogram demonstrating a short-axis view of the carpal tunnel outlet. The thicker transverse carpal ligament (3 *arrows*) is demonstrated.

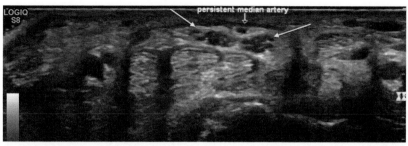

Fig. 20. Sonogram demonstrating a short-axis view of a bifid median nerve (*long arrows* point to median fascicles) with an intervening persistent median artery.

Procedure

a. Needle: 25 gauge, 38 to 51 mm (**Figs. 25** and **26**).[72–74]
b. Patient position: Supine.
c. Transducer position: Short-axis to the nerve, generally in-plane with inguinal ligament.
d. Needle approach: Lateral-to-medial for single injection. Use of lateral-to-medial and also distal-to-proximal for hydrodissection.
e. Target: The area around the nerve at the level of the inguinal ligament and somewhat distal in the space anterior to the fascial plane between the sartorius and tensor fascia lata.
f. Avoid: Deep injections above the inguinal ligament or very medial to the location of the nerve. The nerve is very superficial.

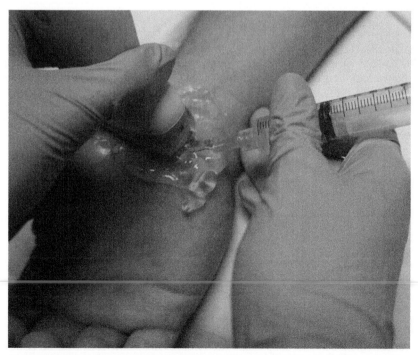

Fig. 21. Arrangement for an injection near the median nerve at the level of the carpal tunnel.

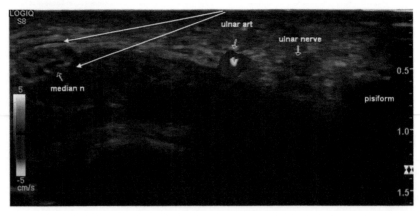

Fig. 22. Sonogram demonstrating the needle approaches (*long arrows*) for an injection near the median nerve in short-axis at the level of the carpal tunnel.

Superficial Fibular (Peroneal) Nerve at the Leg

Indications

The superficial fibular nerve is most frequently injured at the mid-leg where it exits the crural fascia from the lateral compartment and becomes subcutaneous.[75] In most individuals, this occurs 8 to 12 cm proximal to the tip of the lateral malleolus.[76–78] Neuropathy at this location can occur from entrapment in fascia, stretch from an inversion ankle sprain, lateral compartment syndrome, or other trauma.[79–82] Neuropathy of the superficial fibular nerve at this location can result in sensory disturbance and pain in the lateral leg and dorsum of the foot.

Anatomy

The superficial fibular nerve bifurcates from the common fibular nerve in the area of the fibular head. It travels in the lateral compartment and exits between the fibularis longus and brevis and the extensor digitorum (**Fig. 27**). It becomes subcutaneous and traverses distally in the leg. It then divides into lateral and intermediate branches that travel to the dorsum of the foot.[83] It provides motor branches to the fibularis longus and brevis, then continues on to provide cutaneous sensation to the lateral aspect of the leg and dorsum of the foot.

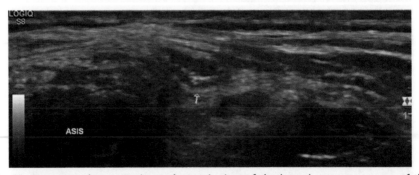

Fig. 23. Sonogram demonstrating a short-axis view of the lateral cutaneous nerve of the thigh (*arrow*) at the level of the inguinal ligament.

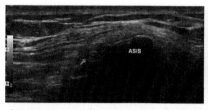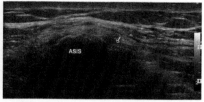

Fig. 24. Sonograms demonstrating short-axis views of the lateral cutaneous nerve of the thigh (*arrows*). The affected side (*left image*) is enlarged and more conspicuous than the asymptomatic side (*right image*).

Scanning

The nerve should be scanned in short-axis and inspected at its exit point from the lateral compartment as well as distal to its branch points. The nerve should be inspected for focal enlargement and signs of fascial defect, muscle herniation, or any other anatomic source of focal neuropathy.[84]

Procedure

a. Needle: 25 gauge, 25 to 38 mm (**Figs. 28** and **29**).
b. Patient position: Supine or lateral decubitus.
c. Transducer position: Short-axis to the nerve. Both short-axis and long-axis often used for hydrodissection.
d. Needle approach: Anterior-to-posterior or posterior-to-lateral for a single injection. Additional approach of distal-to-proximal for hydrodissection.
e. Target: The area around the nerve, often as it exits the crural fascia and becomes subcutaneous.
f. Avoid: Injecting too deep. The nerve is very superficial.

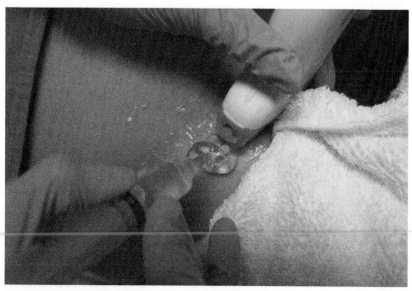

Fig. 25. Arrangement for an injection near the lateral cutaneous nerve of the thigh in short-axis at the level of the inguinal ligament.

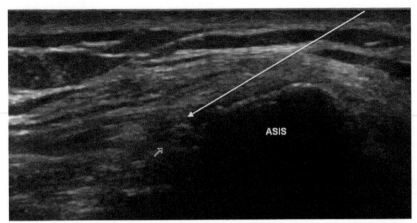

Fig. 26. Sonogram demonstrating the needle approach (*long arrow*) for an injection near the lateral cutaneous nerve of the thigh (*small arrow*) in the area of the ASIS.

Tibial Nerve at the Ankle

Indications

Tibial nerve injections at the ankle are often performed for local anesthesia to reduce pain from procedures at the plantar aspect of the foot. Injections in this area also can be used for suspected tibial neuropathy at the tarsal tunnel. Idiopathic neuropathy in this location with a diagnosis of tarsal tunnel syndrome is somewhat controversial.[85] Regardless, neuropathy can occur as a result of multiple factors, including surrounding tenosynovitis, venous thrombosis, ganglion cysts, encroachment of osteophytes, trauma, and structural foot and ankle deformities.[86,87] Neuropathy at this level can

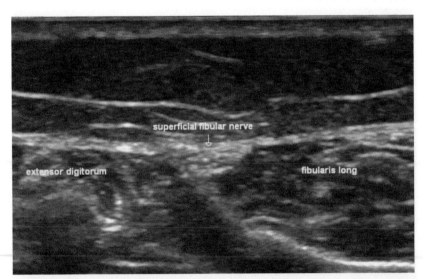

Fig. 27. Sonogram demonstrating a short-axis view of the superficial fibular nerve at the mid-leg near its exit point from the lateral compartment between the extensor digitorum longus and the fibularis longus and brevis.

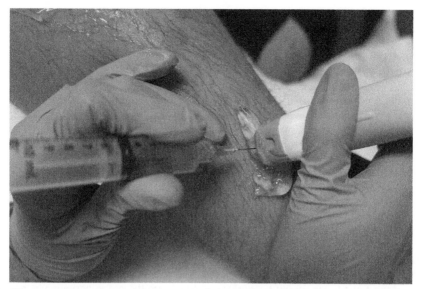

Fig. 28. Arrangement for an injection near the superficial fibular nerve at the mid-leg.

present as medial ankle pain and paresthesias at the plantar aspect of the foot.[88,89] Less commonly, weakness of the foot intrinsic muscles can be seen.[90]

Anatomy

The tibial nerve is derived from the L4, L5, S1, S2, and S3 roots and traverses from the posterior compartment of the leg to the medial ankle and through the tarsal tunnel. The tarsal tunnel is divided into upper (tibiotalar) and lower (talocalcaneal) compartments. The upper compartment is covered by the crural fascia and has an osseous floor that

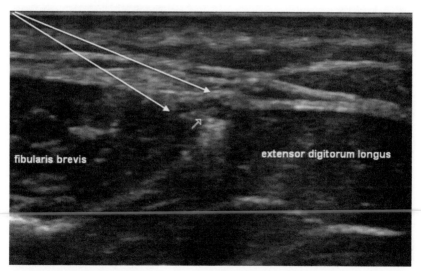

Fig. 29. Sonogram demonstrating the needle approaches (*long arrows*) for an injection near the superficial fibular nerve in short-axis (*small arrow*) at the mid-leg.

is formed by the posterior aspect of the distal tibia and the talus.[91] It contains the tibia-lis posterior tendon, the flexor digitorum longus tendon, posterior tibial artery and veins, tibial nerve, and flexor hallucis longus (**Fig. 30**).

The lower compartment is considered the "true" tarsal tunnel. It is covered by the flexor retinaculum and the abductor hallucis.[92] Its bony floor consists of portions of the talus, sustentaculum tali, and calcaneus.[93] The medial calcaneal branch usually bi-furcates from the main trunk of the tibial nerve before its entrance into the flexor reti-naculum; however, there is considerable individual variation.[94,95] The bifurcation point of the medial and lateral plantar branches also varies, but often becomes distinct in the distal portion of the tarsal tunnel.[96]

Scanning

The tibial nerve should be scanned in short-axis view from the distal leg through the tarsal tunnel space. Particular effort should be made toward recognizing the locations of the branch points of the medial calcaneal nerve, as well as the bifurcation into the medial and lateral plantar nerves (**Fig. 31**). These locations can have implications with the efficacy of an injection. The surrounding anatomy should be surveyed in detail. Assessment of the nerve and surrounding structures also should be performed in long-axis for complete perspective (**Fig. 32**). Sufficient anterior and posterior move-ment of the transducer should be performed to ensure the entire nerve is visualized, particularly distal to the bifurcation points when there is separation of the fascicles. The nerve should be inspected for signs of focal enlargement, notching, change in fascicular architecture, and encroachment by surrounding tissue.[97–99]

Procedure

a. Needle: 22 to 25 gauge, 38 to 51 mm (**Figs. 33** and **34**).
b. Patient position: Lateral decubitus or prone.
c. Transducer position: Short-axis to the nerve.
d. Needle approach: Posterior-to-anterior.

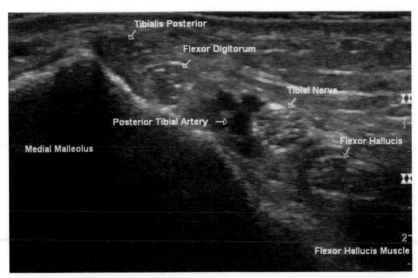

Fig. 30. Sonogram demonstrating a short-axis view of the medial ankle and tarsal tunnel space.

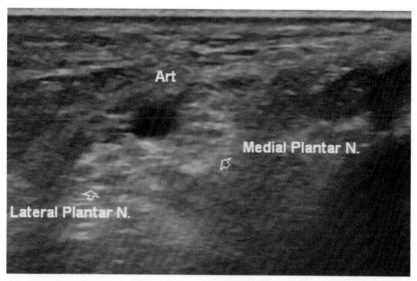

Fig. 31. Sonogram demonstrating a short-axis view of the medial and lateral plantar nerves after bifurcation.

e. Target: The area around the tibial nerve. Care should be taken to target the tibial nerve proximal to the bifurcation of the medial calcaneal branch when anesthetic blocks for plantar foot procedures are being performed.

f. Avoid: Intraneural and intravascular injections. Doppler flow can assist with identifying the vascular structures. Increasing and decreasing transducer pressure can assist with vein identification.

Interdigital Neuroma

Indications

Interdigital neuroma is a fusiform enlargement of one of the common plantar digital nerves. The precise cause is controversial but it is felt to arise from repetitive mechanical irritation resulting in perineural fibrosis and thickening of the nerve; thus, it is not a true neuroma.[100] It can be a source of pain in the distal foot, often in the distribution of the interdigital nerve. Injections into the neuroma may include local anesthetic, corticosteroids, and even sclerosing agents, such as dilute alcohol or radiofrequency ablation.[101–104]

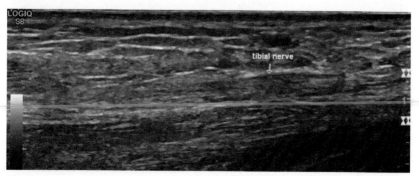

Fig. 32. Sonogram demonstrating a long-axis view of the tibial nerve at the ankle.

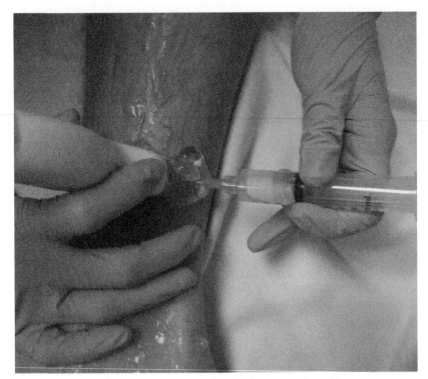

Fig. 33. Arrangement for an injection near the tibial nerve at the ankle.

Anatomy

Interdigital neuroma most often occurs in the third web space and less frequency develops in the second web space. It rarely occurs in the first or fourth web space.[105] The interdigital nerves are extensions of the distal communicating branches of the medial and lateral plantar nerves. They lie inferior to the intermetatarsal ligament at the level of the metatarsal heads.

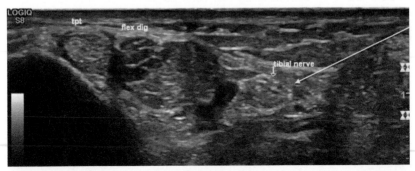

Fig. 34. Sonogram demonstrating the needle approach (*long arrow*) for an injection near the tibial nerve at the ankle. The tibialis posterior tendon (tpt) and flexor digitorum tendon (flex dig) are shown.

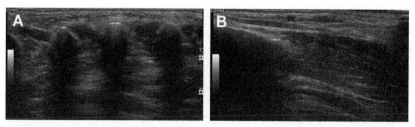

Fig. 35. Sonograms demonstrating the short-axis (*A*) and long-axis (*B*) views of the intermetatarsal space.

Scanning

Ultrasound has good accuracy for identification and measurement of interdigital neuromas.[106–108] The transducer is scanned over the distal metatarsal region, usually in short-axis at first, but is also compared in long-axis (**Fig. 35**). The foot can be examined from both the dorsal and plantar aspects. Caution should be used to maintain correct orientation when alternating scanning directions. Dynamic compression while imaging with ultrasound can be helpful in distinguishing an interdigital neuroma from intermetatarsal bursitis. The neuroma appears as a slightly irregular hypoechoic mass in the intermetatarsal space, plantar to the intermetatarsal ligament.[109] With transducer pressure, an intermetatarsal bursitis will compress and an interdigital neuroma will not. The area also should be assessed for bone irregularity and surrounding synovitis.

Procedure

a. Needle: 25 to 27 gauge, 38 mm (**Figs. 36** and **37**).[2]
b. Patient position: Prone or supine.
c. Transducer position: Long-axis between the metatarsal heads after initially scanning in short-axis.
d. Needle approach: Distal-to-proximal approaching from the web space.

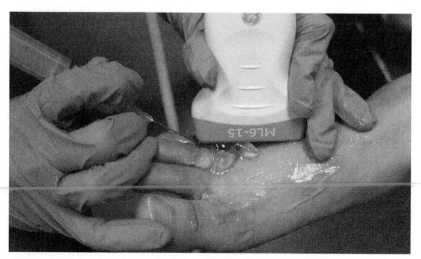

Fig. 36. Arrangement for an interdigital neuroma injection.

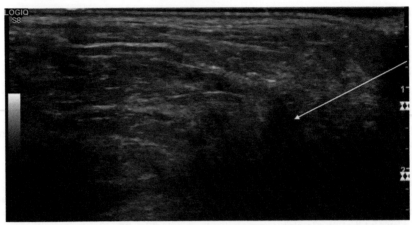

Fig. 37. Sonogram demonstrating the needle approach (*long arrow*) for an interdigital neuroma injection. The transducer is placed in long-axis in the intermetatarsal space and the needle is directed in-plane from the more distal web space to the hypoechoic neuroma.

   e. Target: Around and into the neuroma.
   f. Avoid: Direct injection of the digital arteries.

SUMMARY

Ultrasound guidance allows real-time visualization of the needle in peripheral nerve procedures with improved accuracy and safety. The visualization of the vulnerable target of the peripheral nerve as well as surrounding anatomy can provide valuable information for both diagnostic purposes and procedure enhancement. Detailed knowledge of anatomy and appropriate preprocedural scanning and equipment preparation can facilitate effective use of ultrasound guidance for peripheral nerve procedures.

REFERENCES

1. Jacobson JA. Fundamentals of musculoskeletal ultrasound. 2nd edition. Philadelphia: Elsevier Saunders; 2013.
2. Malanga G, Mautner K. Atlas of ultrasound-guided musculoskeletal injections. New York: McGraw-Hill; 2013.
3. Bigeleisen PE. Nerve puncture and apparent intraneural injection during ultrasound-guided axillary block does not invariably result in neurologic injury. Anesthesiology 2006;105(4):779–83.
4. Jeng CL, Torrillo TM, Rosenblatt MA. Complications of peripheral nerve blocks. Br J Anaesth 2010;105(Suppl 1):i97–107.
5. Jeng CL, Rosenblatt MA. Intraneural injections and regional anesthesia: the known and the unknown. Minerva Anestesiol 2011;77(1):54–8.
6. Choquet O, Morau D, Biboulet P, et al. Where should the tip of the needle be located in ultrasound-guided peripheral nerve blocks? Curr Opin Anaesthesiol 2012;25(5):596–602.
7. Dufour E, Donat N, Jaziri S, et al. Ultrasound-guided perineural circumferential median nerve block with and without prior dextrose 5% hydrodissection: a prospective randomized double-blinded noninferiority trial. Anesth Analg 2012; 115(3):728–33.

8. Strakowski JA. Introduction to musculoskeletal ultrasound: getting started. New York: Demos Medical Publishing; 2016.

9. Lento PA, Strakowski JA. The use of ultrasound in guiding musculoskeletal interventional procedures. Phys Med Rehabil Clin N Am 2010;21:559–83.

10. Mulvaney SW. Ultrasound-guided percutaneous neuroplasty of the lateral femoral cutaneous nerve for the treatment of meralgia paresthetica: a case report and description of a new ultrasound-guided technique. Curr Sports Med Rep 2011;10(2):99–104.

11. Fader RR, Mitchell JJ, Chadayammuri VP, et al. Percutaneous ultrasound-guided hydrodissection of a symptomatic sural neuroma. Orthopedics 2015; 38(11):e1046–50.

12. Cass SP. Ultrasound-guided nerve hydrodissection: what is it? A review of the literature. Curr Sports Med Rep 2016;15(1):20–2.

13. Siegenthaler A, Moriggl B, Mlekusch S, et al. Ultrasound-guided suprascapular nerve block, description of a novel supraclavicular approach. Reg Anesth Pain Med 2012;37(3):325–8.

14. Liveson JA, Bronson MJ, Pollack MA. Suprascapular nerve lesions at the spinoglenoid notch: report of three cases and review of the literature. J Neurol Neurosurg Psychiatry 1991;54(3):241–3.

15. Hashimoto BE, Hayes AS, Ager JD. Sonographic diagnosis and treatment of ganglion cysts causing suprascapular nerve entrapment. J Ultrasound Med 1994;13(9):671–4.

16. Rachbauer F, Sterzinger W, Frischhut B. Suprascapular nerve entrapment at the spinoglenoid notch caused by a ganglion cyst. J Shoulder Elbow Surg 1996;5(2 Pt 1):150–2.

17. Chiou HJ, Chou YH, Wu JJ, et al. Alternative and effective treatment of shoulder ganglion cyst: ultrasonographically guided aspiration. J Ultrasound Med 1999; 18(8):531–5.

18. Duparc F, Coquerel D, Ozeel J, et al. Anatomical basis of the suprascapular nerve entrapment, and clinical relevance of the supraspinatus fascia. Surg Radiol Anat 2010;32(3):277–84.

19. Safran MR. Nerve injury about the shoulder in athletes, part 1: suprascapular nerve and axillary nerve. Am J Sports Med 2004;32(3):803–19.

20. Martinoli C, Bianchi S, Prato N, et al. US of the shoulder: non-rotator cuff disorders. Radiographics 2003;23:381.

21. Martinoli C, Bianchi S, Pugliese F, et al. Sonography of entrapment neuropathies in the upper limb (wrist excluded). J Clin Ultrasound 2004;32(9):438–50.

22. Peng PW, Wiley MJ, Liang J, et al. Ultrasound-guided suprascapular nerve block: a correlation with fluoroscopic and cadaveric findings. Can J Anaesth 2010;57(2):143–8.

23. Harmon D, Hearty C. Ultrasound-guided suprascapular nerve block technique. Pain Physician 2007;10(6):743–6.

24. Chan CW, Peng PW. Suprascapular nerve block: a narrative review. Reg Anesth Pain Med 2011;36(4):358–73.

25. Roles NC, Maudsley RH. Radial tunnel syndrome: resistant tennis elbow as a nerve entrapment. J Bone Joint Surg Br 1972;54(3):499–508.

26. Rosenbaum R. Disputed radial tunnel syndrome. Muscle Nerve 1999;22(7): 960–7.

27. Stanley J. Radial tunnel syndrome: a surgeon's perspective. J Hand Ther 2006; 19(2):180–4.

28. Stöhr M. Does the algetic supinator syndrome exist? Handchir Mikrochir Plast Chir 2009;41(1):35–7.
29. Ozturk A, Kutlu C, Taskara N, et al. Anatomic and morphometric study of the arcade of Frohse in cadavers. Surg Radiol Anat 2005;27(3):171–5.
30. Hazani R, Engineer NJ, Mowlavi A, et al. Anatomic landmarks for the radial tunnel. Eplasty 2008;8:e37.
31. Hill S, Hall S. Microscopic anatomy of the posterior interosseous and median nerves at sites of potential entrapment in the forearm. J Hand Surg Br 1999; 24(2):170–6.
32. Lubahn JD, Cermak MB. Uncommon nerve compression syndromes of the upper extremity. J Am Acad Orthop Surg 1998;6(6):378–86.
33. Fuss FK. The eponym of the supinator arch. Surg Radiol Anat 1996;18(2):158.
34. Weinstein SM, Herring SA. Nerve problems and compartment syndromes in the hand, wrist, and forearm. Clin Sports Med 1992;11(1):161–88.
35. Lawrence T, Mobbs P, Fortems Y, et al. Radial tunnel syndrome. A retrospective review of 30 decompressions of the radial nerve. J Hand Surg Br 1995;20(4): 454–9.
36. Clavert P, Lutz JC, Adam P, et al. Frohse's arcade is not the exclusive compression site of the radial nerve in its tunnel. Orthop Traumatol Surg Res 2009;95(2): 114–8.
37. Bodner G, Harpf C, Meirer R, et al. Ultrasonographic appearance of supinator syndrome. J Ultrasound Med 2002;21(11):1289–93.
38. Strakowski JA. Ultrasound evaluation of focal neuropathies. Correlation with electrodiagnosis. New York: Demos Medical; 2014.
39. Meng S, Tinhofer I, Weninger WJ, et al. Ultrasound and anatomical correlation of the radial nerve at the arcade of Frohse. Muscle Nerve 2015;51(6):853–8.
40. Rodner CM, Tinsley BA, O'Malley MP. Pronator syndrome and anterior interosseous nerve syndrome. J Am Acad Orthop Surg 2013;21(5):268–75.
41. Wertsch JJ, Melvin J. Median nerve anatomy and entrapment syndromes: a review. Arch Phys Med Rehabil 1982;63(12):623–7.
42. Carter GT, Weiss MD. Diagnosis and treatment of work-related proximal median and radial nerve entrapment. Phys Med Rehabil Clin N Am 2015;26(3):539–49.
43. Kowalska B, Sudoł-Szopińska I. Ultrasound assessment on selected peripheral nerve pathologies. Part I: entrapment neuropathies of the upper limb— excluding carpal tunnel syndrome. J Ultrason 2012;12(50):307–18.
44. Jacobson JA, Fessell DP, Lobo Lda G, et al. Entrapment neuropathies I: upper limb (carpal tunnel excluded). Semin Musculoskelet Radiol 2010;14(5):473–86.
45. Lee J, Lee YS. Percutaneous chemical nerve block with ultrasound-guided intraneural injection. Eur Radiol 2008;18(7):1506–12.
46. Loong SC. The carpal tunnel syndrome: a clinical and electrophysiological study of 250 patients. Clin Exp Neurol 1977;14:51–65.
47. El Miedany YM, Aty SA, Ashour S. Ultrasonography versus nerve conduction study in patients with carpal tunnel syndrome: substantive or complementary tests? Rheumatology (Oxford) 2004;43(7):887–95.
48. Kaymak B, Ozçakar L, Cetin A, et al. A comparison of the benefits of sonography and electrophysiologic measurements as predictors of symptom severity and functional status in patients with carpal tunnel syndrome. Arch Phys Med Rehabil 2008;89(4):743–8.
49. Moran L, Perez M, Esteban A, et al. Sonographic measurement of cross-sectional area of the median nerve in the diagnosis of carpal tunnel syndrome: correlation with nerve conduction studies. J Clin Ultrasound 2009;37(3):125–31.

50. Cartwright MS, White DL, Demar S, et al. Median nerve changes following steroid injection for carpal tunnel syndrome. Muscle Nerve 2011;44(1):25–9.
51. Netter FH. Atlas of human anatomy. 3rd edition. New Jersey: Icon Learning Systems; 2003.
52. Kamolz LP, Schrögendorfer KF, Rab M, et al. The precision of ultrasound imaging and its relevance for carpal tunnel syndrome. Surg Radiol Anat 2001;23(2): 117–21.
53. Wiesler ER, Chloros GD, Cartwright MS, et al. The use of diagnostic ultrasound in carpal tunnel syndrome. J Hand Surg Am 2006;31(5):726–32.
54. Peetrons PA, Derbali W. Carpal tunnel syndrome. Semin Musculoskelet Radiol 2013;17(1):28–33.
55. Jamadar DA, Jacobson JA, Hayes CW. Sonographic evaluation of the median nerve at the wrist. J Ultrasound Med 2001;20(9):1011–4.
56. Sarría L, Cabada T, Cozcolluela R, et al. Carpal tunnel syndrome: usefulness of sonography. Eur Radiol 2000;10(12):1920–5.
57. Yu G, Chen Q, Wang D, et al. Diagnosis of carpal tunnel syndrome assessed using high-frequency ultrasonography: cross-section areas of 8-site median nerve. Clin Rheumatol 2016. [Epub ahead of print].
58. Propeck T, Quinn TJ, Jacobson JA, et al. Sonography and MR imaging of bifid median nerve with anatomic and histologic correlation. AJR Am J Roentgenol 2000;175(6):1721–5.
59. Bayrak IK, Bayrak AO, Kale M, et al. Bifid median nerve in patients with carpal tunnel syndrome. J Ultrasound Med 2008;27(8):1129–36.
60. Lisanti M, Rosati M, Pardi A. Persistent median artery in carpal tunnel syndrome. Acta Orthop Belg 1995;61(4):315–8.
61. Racasan O, Dubert T. The safest location for steroid injection in the treatment of carpal tunnel syndrome. J Hand Surg Br 2005;30(4):412–4.
62. Smith J, Wisniewski SJ, Finnoff JT, et al. Sonographically guided carpal tunnel injections: the ulnar approach. J Ultrasound Med 2008;27(10):1485–90.
63. Lee JY, Park Y, Park KD, et al. Effectiveness of ultrasound-guided carpal tunnel injection using in-plane ulnar approach: a prospective, randomized, single-blinded study. Medicine (Baltimore) 2014;93(29):e350.
64. Patijn J, Mekhail N, Hayek S, et al. Meralgia paresthetica. Pain Pract 2011;11(3): 302–8.
65. Grossman MG, Ducey SA, Nadler SS, et al. Meralgia paresthetica: diagnosis and treatment. J Am Acad Orthop Surg 2001;9(5):336–44.
66. Corujo A, Franco CD, Williams JM. The sensory territory of the lateral cutaneous nerve of the thigh as determined by anatomic dissections and ultrasound-guided blocks. Reg Anesth Pain Med 2012;37(5):561–4.
67. de Ridder VA, de Lange S, Popta JV. Anatomical variations of the lateral femoral cutaneous nerve and the consequences for surgery. J Orthop Trauma 1999; 13(3):207–11.
68. Carai A, Fenu G, Sechi E, et al. Anatomical variability of the lateral femoral cutaneous nerve: findings from a surgical series. Clin Anat 2009;22(3):365–70.
69. Ng I, Vaghadia H, Choi PT, et al. Ultrasound imaging accurately identifies the lateral femoral cutaneous nerve. Anesth Analg 2008;107(3):1070–4.
70. Bodner G, Bernathova M, Galiano K, et al. Ultrasound of the lateral femoral cutaneous nerve: normal findings in a cadaver and in volunteers. Reg Anesth Pain Med 2009;34(3):265–8.
71. Damarey B, Demondion X, Boutry N, et al. Sonographic assessment of the lateral femoral cutaneous nerve. J Clin Ultrasound 2009;37(2):89–95.

72. Hurdle MF, Weingarten TN, Crisostomo RA, et al. Ultrasound-guided blockade of the lateral femoral cutaneous nerve: technical description and review of 10 cases. Arch Phys Med Rehabil 2007;88(10):1362–4.

73. Tumber PS, Bhatia A, Chan VW. Ultrasound-guided lateral femoral cutaneous nerve block for meralgia paresthetica. Anesth Analg 2008;106(3):1021–2.

74. Tagliafico A, Serafini G, Lacelli F, et al. Ultrasound-guided treatment of meralgia paresthetica (lateral femoral cutaneous neuropathy): technical description and results of treatment in 20 consecutive patients. J Ultrasound Med 2011; 30(10):1341–6.

75. Ribak S, Fonseca JR, Tietzmann A, et al. The anatomy and morphology of the superficial peroneal nerve. J Reconstr Microsurg 2015;32(4):271–5.

76. Pacha D, Carrera A, Llusa M, et al. Clinical anatomy of the superficial peroneal nerve in the distal leg. Eur J Anat 2003;7(Suppl 1):15–20.

77. Ucerler H, Ikiz A. The variations of the sensory branches of the superficial peroneal nerve course and its clinical importance. Foot Ankle Int 2005;26(11):942–6.

78. Prakash, Bhardwaj AK, Singh DK, et al. Anatomic variations of superficial peroneal nerve: clinical implications of a cadaver study. Ital J Anat Embryol 2010; 115(3):223–8.

79. McAuliffe TB, Fiddian NJ, Browett JP. Entrapment neuropathy of the superficial peroneal nerve. A bilateral case. J Bone Joint Surg Br 1985;67(1):62–3.

80. Styf J. Entrapment of the superficial peroneal nerve. Diagnosis and results of decompression. J Bone Joint Surg Br 1989;71(1):131–5.

81. Ogüt T, Akgün I, Kesmezacar H, et al. Navigation for ankle arthroscopy: anatomical study of the anterolateral portal with reference to the superficial peroneal nerve. Surg Radiol Anat 2004;26(4):268–74.

82. Yang LJ, Gala VC, McGillicuddy JE. Superficial peroneal nerve syndrome: an unusual nerve entrapment. Case report. J Neurosurg 2006;104(5):820–3.

83. Blair JM, Botte MJ. Surgical anatomy of the superficial peroneal nerve in the ankle and foot. Clin Orthop Relat Res 1994;305:229–38.

84. Canella C, Demondion X, Guillin R, et al. Anatomic study of the superficial peroneal nerve using sonography. AJR Am J Roentgenol 2009;193(1):174–9.

85. Dawson DM, Hallett M, Wilbourn AJ. Entrapment neuropathies. 3rd edition. Philadelphia (NY): Lippincott-Raven; 1999.

86. Erickson SJ, Quinn SF, Kneeland JB, et al. MR imaging of the tarsal tunnel and related spaces: normal and abnormal findings with anatomic correlation. AJR Am J Roentgenol 1990;155(2):323–8.

87. Fantino O, Coillard JY, Borne J, et al. Ultrasound of the tarsal tunnel: normal and pathological imaging features. J Radiol 2011;92(12):1072–80 [in French].

88. Schon LC. Nerve entrapment, neuropathy, and nerve dysfunction in athletes. Orthop Clin North Am 1994;25(1):47–59.

89. Kwok KB, Lui TH, Lo WN. Neurilemmoma of the first branch of the lateral plantar nerve causing tarsal tunnel syndrome. Foot Ankle Spec 2009;2(6):287–90.

90. Goodgold J, Kopell HP, Spielholz NI. The tarsal-tunnel syndrome. Objective diagnostic criteria. N Engl J Med 1965;273(14):742–5.

91. Finkel JE. Tarsal tunnel syndrome. Magn Reson Imaging Clin N Am 1994;2(1): 67–78.

92. Zeiss J, Fenton P, Ebraheim N, et al. Normal magnetic resonance anatomy of the tarsal tunnel. Foot Ankle 1990;10(4):214–8.

93. Martinoli C, Court-Payen M, Michaud J, et al. Imaging of neuropathies about the ankle and foot. Semin Musculoskelet Radiol 2010;14(3):344–56.

94. Dellon AL, Mackinnon SE. Tibial nerve branching in the tarsal tunnel. Arch Neurol 1984;41(6):645–6.
95. Davis TJ, Schon LC. Branches of the tibial nerve: anatomic variations. Foot Ankle Int 1995;16(1):21–9.
96. Havel PE, Ebraheim NA, Clark SE, et al. Tibial nerve branching in the tarsal tunnel. Foot Ankle 1988;9(3):117–9.
97. Machiels F, Shahabpour M, De Maeseneer M, et al. Tarsal tunnel syndrome: ultrasonographic and MRI features. JBR-BTR 1999;82(2):49–50.
98. Kinoshita M, Okuda R, Morikawa J, et al. Tarsal tunnel syndrome associated with an accessory muscle. Foot Ankle Int 2003;24(2):132–6.
99. Vijayan J, Therimadasamy AK, Teoh HL, et al. Sonography as an aid to neurophysiological studies in diagnosing tarsal tunnel syndrome. Am J Phys Med Rehabil 2009;88(6):500–1.
100. Kim JY, Choi JH, Park J, et al. An anatomical study of Morton's interdigital neuroma: the relationship between the occurring site and the deep transverse metatarsal ligament (DTML). Foot Ankle Int 2007;28(9):1007–10.
101. Markovic M, Crichton K, Read JW, et al. Effectiveness of ultrasound-guided corticosteroid injection in the treatment of Morton's neuroma. Foot Ankle Int 2008;29(5):483–7.
102. Makki D, Haddad BZ, Mahmood Z, et al. Efficacy of corticosteroid injection versus size of plantar interdigital neuroma. Foot Ankle Int 2012;33(9):722–6.
103. Chuter GS, Chua YP, Connell DA, et al. Ultrasound-guided radiofrequency ablation in the management of interdigital (Morton's) neuroma. Skeletal Radiol 2013;42(1):107–11.
104. Pasquali C, Vulcano E, Novario R, et al. Ultrasound-guided alcohol injection for Morton's neuroma. Foot Ankle Int 2015;36(1):55–9.
105. Redd RA, Peters VJ, Emery SF, et al. Morton neuroma: sonographic evaluation. Radiology 1989;171:415–7.
106. Sobiesk GA, Wertheimer SJ, Schulz R, et al. Sonographic evaluation of interdigital neuromas. J Foot Ankle Surg 1997;36(5):364–6.
107. Read JW, Noakes JB, Kerr D, et al. Morton's metatarsalgia: sonographic findings and correlated histopathology. Foot Ankle Int 1999;20(3):153–61.
108. Shapiro PP, Shapiro SL. Sonographic evaluation of interdigital neuromas. Foot Ankle Int 1995;16(10):604–6.
109. Lee MJ, Kim S, Huh YM, et al. Morton neuroma: evaluated with ultrasonography and MR imaging. Korean J Radiol 2007;8(2):148–55.

Orthobiologic Interventions Using Ultrasound Guidance

Gerard Malanga, MD[a,b,*], Dena Abdelshahed, MD[a], Prathap Jayaram, MD[c]

KEYWORDS

- Platelet-rich plasma • Stem cell therapy • Orthobiologics • Biologic agents
- Regenerative medicine • Tendon • Ligament • Muscle

KEY POINTS

- Regenerative medicine techniques, including platelet-rich plasma (PRP) and mesenchymal stem cell (MSC) therapy, are becoming increasingly popular for the treatment of surgical and nonsurgical musculoskeletal injuries.
- PRP and MSCs, collectively referred to as orthobiologics, work by augmenting natural healing processes and have been found effective at increasing tissue regeneration.
- Orthobiologics are becoming increasingly preferred over conventional treatments, including anti-inflammatory medications and corticosteroid injections, which have been shown to have adverse effects.
- Ultrasound guidance can assist in the performance of the various procedures used in regenerative medicine, ranging from venipuncture to bone marrow and adipose aspiration.
- Further high-quality research on PRP and MSCs will serve to further define the most appropriate and effective applications for these treatments.

INTRODUCTION

Historical and recent evidence increasingly refute the use of corticosteroid injections for most sports injuries, especially tendinopathies. Coombes and colleagues[1,2] studied lateral epicondylalgia and found poorer long-term outcomes with local corticosteroid injections compared with placebo. The application of regenerative therapies for the

Disclosures: None.
[a] Department of Physical Medicine and Rehabilitation, Rutgers University-New Jersey Medical School, Newark, NJ, USA; [b] New Jersey Regenerative Institute, 197 Ridgedale Avenue, Suite 210, Cedar Knolls, NJ 07927, USA; [c] Department of Physical Medicine and Rehabilitation, Baylor College of Medicine, Houston, TX, USA
* Corresponding author. New Jersey Regenerative Institute, 197 Ridgedale Avenue, Suite 210, Cedar Knolls, NJ 07927.
E-mail address: gmalangamd@hotmail.com

Phys Med Rehabil Clin N Am 27 (2016) 717–731
http://dx.doi.org/10.1016/j.pmr.2016.04.007
1047-9651/16/$ – see front matter © 2016 Elsevier Inc. All rights reserved.

treatment of musculoskeletal conditions has emerged over the last decade with recent acceleration. These include prolotherapy, platelet-rich plasma (PRP), and mesenchymal stem cell (MSC) therapy. In brief, these strategies augment the body's innate physiology to heal pathologic processes. This article focuses on some of the specific issues related to PRP and adipose and bone marrow MSC procedures, often collectively referred to as orthobiologics. Discussed are issues related to PRP and MSC injection procedures not addressed elsewhere in this issue. We also review specific factors related to patient and target tissue selection for the use of biologic agents for tendon, ligament, joint, and spinal pathologies.

PLATELET-RICH PLASMA
Background

Wound healing naturally occurs in three phases: (1) the inflammatory phase, (2) the proliferative phase, and (3) the remodeling phase. Platelets, nonnucleated blood components formed from megakaryocytes, play an integral role in this process.[3] Alpha granules within platelets include many growth factors, including insulin-like growth factor 1, platelet-derived growth factor, vascular endothelial growth factor, and transforming growth factor (TGF)-β1.[4] These growth factors, among others released by platelets, influence chemotaxis and induce angiogenesis and extracellular matrix production, eventually leading to tissue repair.[5]

Definition

PRP is autologous blood containing a higher than physiologic concentration of platelets.[6] Considering this definition, no two samples of PRP are identical. The efficacy of PRP is therefore likely impacted by the composition of the PRP itself. It is challenging to compare the efficacy of PRP across clinical studies if the composition of the PRP used is not reported in detail. Several classification systems for PRP have been proposed, although none have been widely accepted.[7–10] The Platelet Count, Leukocyte Presence, Red Blood Cell Presence, and Use of Activation classification system identifies PRP samples by platelet concentration (absolute number of platelets), leukocyte concentration (including concentration of neutrophils), red blood cell concentration, and activation by exogenous agents.[11] This classification has been suggested as more specifically categorizing the type of PRP injected especially when reported in clinical studies.

Mechanism of Action

The concept supporting the clinical use of PRP is the augmentation of healing processes in tissues with low intrinsic healing potential.[3] Several studies have investigated the mechanism in which this occurs. Kajikawa and colleagues[12] found that PRP activated circulation-derived cells (which play an important role in the healing processes of tissues) in wounded rat patellar tendons. PRP has also been shown to increase levels of growth factors that promote angiogenesis, increasing the blood supply to the injured area. This then allows for circulating factors to reach the injured area to promote healing and remodeling.[5]

Growth factors in PRP also give it anabolic properties; it increases tenocyte proliferation, matrix gene expression, protein production, and chemotaxis of bone marrow cells. Furthermore, TGF-β1, found in PRP, inhibits the expression and release of multiple catabolic growth factors including interleukin (IL)-1β and tumor necrosis factor (TNF)-α. The anti-inflammatory effects of PRP are evident in its use in osteoarthritis (OA). It was found to decrease expression of nuclear factor kappa-light-chain-enhancer of activated B cells, a major inflammation regulator.[13]

A PRP injection usually requires 60 to 100 mL of whole blood obtained via peripheral venipuncture. The whole blood undergoes processing as described later for PRP to be harvested. Although peripheral venipuncture is most often done in other settings without imaging guidance, it is challenging for clinicians who do not otherwise routinely perform venipuncture in their practice. Ultrasound guidance is commonly used during the placement of central venous catheters in emergency department and intensive care unit settings. However, recent studies have also found benefit of ultrasound guidance in small vessel, peripheral venous access.[14]

Peripheral veins can often be visualized (in patients with fair skin or prominent veins) or palpated. Deeper veins are difficult to identify without imaging guidance and thus can be more difficult to access. Ultrasound guidance has been shown to increase overall success of peripheral venous catheterization while decreasing time needed for cannulation. Another important factor to consider is the number of skin punctures or attempts needed to catheterize a vein. Multiple skin punctures increase the risk of complications (infection and bleeding) and patient discomfort. Ultrasound guidance provides the advantage of a higher likelihood of successful venous access on the first attempt.[14]

When using ultrasound guidance to assist in venipuncture for PRP, veins of the forearm are used. Veins can be differentiated from arteries using color or power Doppler imaging. Also, veins are easily compressible with probe pressure, whereas arteries are less compressible. Nerves often travel along blood vessels; thus, ultrasound may assist the operator in avoiding nerves and other adjacent structures during venipuncture. The vein is usually visualized in a transverse view, "out of plane" to the approaching needle. With this view, the ultrasound operator can visualize the tip of the needle as it approaches the lumen of the vein (**Figs. 1** and **2**). Given the relatively large volume of

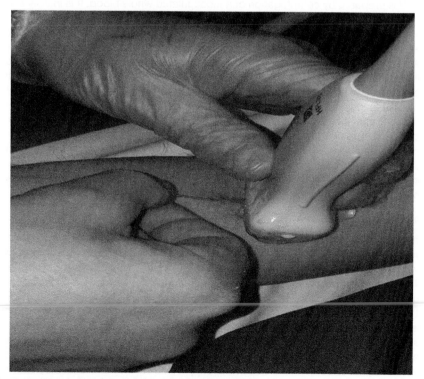

Fig. 1. Approach for ultrasound-guided venipuncture.

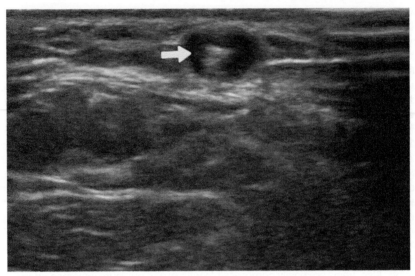

Fig. 2. Ultrasound appearance of needle tip (*arrow*) visualized out-of-plane in the lumen of a vein.

blood needed, ultrasound visualization is maintained throughout the blood draw to ensure the needle stays within the lumen of the vein.

PRP is prepared by centrifugation of anticoagulated whole blood. It is initially separated into three layers based on specific gravity: (1) plasma (top layer), (2) platelets and leukocytes (middle layer, termed the "buffy coat"), and (3) red blood cells (bottom layer). The bottom layer is typically discarded; the buffy coat and top layer are then often subjected to a second centrifugation to separate PRP from platelet-poor plasma. PRP may then be activated with calcium chloride or thrombin to cause the release of growth factors from alpha granules to occur more rapidly, although this additional step is not universally performed. The senior author does not recommend activation with the addition of an agent, but rather natural activation of platelets through contact with degenerative tissue during subsequent injection. Different harvesting and centrifugation kits yield different volumes and concentrations of platelets.[3] It has even been shown that PRP samples produced from the same patient, using the same centrifugation protocol and equipment, may lead to PRP of varying composition.[15]

Evidence for its Application

Although there has been an overall increase in the application of and research regarding the use of PRP, there is still a paucity of randomized control trials producing Level 1 evidence. Lateral epicondylosis is an overuse injury, which in the past was typically treated with a corticosteroid injection. Although there may be inflammation acutely, in chronic tendon injury, there is generally no evidence of inflammatory cells but rather degenerative changes within the tendon. Therefore, the use of anti-inflammatory agents, such as corticosteroids, becomes less logical, and furthermore, has been shown to be harmful to the tendon and clinical outcomes.[2] In contrast, the use of such agents as PRP to stimulate tissue healing would seem to be a more reasonable choice. The current literature seems to support the efficacy of PRP in the treatment of chronic injuries. A comprehensive review of the scientific evidence of PRP for the treatment of all tendinopathies and OA is beyond the scope of this article and has recently been reviewed by Malanga and Nakamura.[16] The authors concluded that there is currently Level 1 evidence to support the use of PRP for treatment of tendinopathies of the elbow and OA of the knee. Additional studies seem to demonstrate efficacy in other tendons and ligaments, although Level 1 evidence is lacking for the use of PRP for the treatment of muscle strain, acute ligamentous sprains, patellar tendinosis, Achilles tendinosis, and rotator cuff injuries, and the authors additionally suggest that additional investigation is needed for the use of PRP in these conditions.[16]

MESENCHYMAL STEM CELLS
Background

MSCs are found abundantly in adipose tissue and bone marrow, and have been used for orthopedic applications given their therapeutic effects that potentiate tissue healing. Their use for clinically relevant therapies has evolved, particularly in musculoskeletal medicine, including cartilage disorders and soft tissue injuries.[17–24]

Definition

Adult MSCs are derived from perivascular cells called pericytes.[17,18] Once a free pericyte, dissociated from the basal lamina of a blood vessel, it is exposed to the chemotactic profile of the soft tissue environment and becomes an MSC.[25] The Mesenchymal and Tissue Stem Cell Committee of the International Society for Cellular Therapy has proposed three criteria to define MSCs: (1) MSCs must be plastic adherent when maintained in standard culture conditions; (2) they must express CD105, CD73, and CD90 and lack expression of CD34, CD45, CD14 or CD11b, CD79a or CD19, and HLA-DR in culture; and (3) MSCs must have the potential to differentiate into osteoblasts, adipocytes, and chondrocytes in vitro.[26]

Mechanism of Action

MSCs have multiple mechanisms that include anti-inflammatory, immunomodulatory, and paracrine effects. In an inflammatory environment that includes IL-1, IL-2, IL-12, TNF-α, and interferon (INF)-γ, MSCs secrete an array of growth factors and anti-inflammatory proteins with complex feedback mechanisms among the many types of immune cells.[27–32] The key immunomodulatory cytokines include prostaglandin E_2, TGF-β1, hepatocyte growth factor, stromal cell-derived factor 1, nitrous oxide, indoleamine 2,3-dioxygenase, IL-4, IL-6, IL-10, IL-1 receptor antagonist, and soluble TNF-α receptor.[28,30,31]

MSCs inhibit many inflammatory cells including T cells, natural killer cells, B cells, monocytes, macrophages, and dendritic cells.[30–34] MSCs promote the transition of T-helper 1 to T-helper 2 cells by reducing INF-γ and increasing IL-4 and IL-10.[35] The restored T-helper 1/T-helper 2 balance has been shown to improve tissue regeneration in cartilage, muscle, and other injuries.[36–41] Reducing INF-γ and production of IL-4 promotes macrophage conversion from M1 (encourage inflammation) to M2 (decrease inflammation). This transition promotes a shift from proinflammatory, antiangiogenic, tissue growth inhibition to anti-inflammatory, proremodeling, and tissue healing.[38,39] The paracrine behavior of secreted bioactive growth factors, cytokines, and chemokines is responsible for the many functions of the MSC immune response and healing potential.[42]

Evidence for Mesenchymal Stem Cell Therapies

Osteoarthritis

The anti-inflammatory and immunomodulator properties of MSCs make them effective in the treatment of articular cartilage defects. A case study done by Goldring[43] demonstrated this regenerative potential examining the use of MSCs in a patient with meniscus and cartilage injuries. Twenty-four weeks after percutaneous injection into the affected knee joint, there was a significant increase in cartilage and meniscus volume, as seen on MRI. The patient attained increased range of motion and decreased pain scores. In addition, several pilot studies have demonstrated improved patient pain scores and functional status after cartilage defect treatment with cultured bone marrow stromal cells.[44] Emadedin and colleagues[45] studied six women who were candidates for joint arthroplasty. They underwent cultured bone marrow MSC injection. MRI in three of the six patients demonstrated decreased edematous subchondral patches. Initial improvements in pain and function were reported; however, 6 months postinjection, all patients presented with recurring pain.

An institutional review board approved registry (Regenexx, IORG0002115) was started in 2005 and is currently collecting outcome and adverse effects data from more than 2500 patients who have received bone marrow concentrate (BMC) injection treatment of various orthopedic conditions. Preliminary, unpublished data collected from 539 cases of BMC application in the knee demonstrate positive results. Of the patients who have returned for follow-up to date (145 patients at 1 month, 98 patients at 1 year, 30 patients at 2 years, and 11 patients at 3 years), improvement in symptoms was demonstrated in 40%, 52%, 60%, and 68%, respectively (J.R. Schultz, unpublished data, 2014).

Sampson and colleagues[46] reported preliminary data with favorable outcomes in 125 patients receiving hip, knee, shoulder, ankle, or cervical zygapophyseal joint BMC injections. There was a 71% reduction in overall pain at a median follow-up of 148 days postinjection in patients with complete data available. When comparing data from 87 patients with both preprocedural and postprocedural pain scores (complete) versus 38 patients with incomplete data, there was no evidence of selection bias, because both groups had similar characteristics (ie, age, body mass index, follow-up time, satisfaction). Knee injections had the largest improvement in pain scores compared with the other joints. Satisfaction with the procedure was reported by 92% of patients, and 95% would recommend the procedure to a friend. Contrary to prior reports in the literature, age had no correlation with outcomes in this cohort of patients; those aged up to 79 years reported positive results. BMC therapy has also been used as an adjunct postoperatively to accelerate healing after procedures, such as arthroscopic debridement, meniscal transplantation, and subchondroplasty.[46]

Adipose-derived MSCs have also shown clinical promise. Koh and Choi[47] performed MSC injection in conjunction with arthroscopic lavage in elderly patients with knee OA. Two years later, 14 of the 16 patients underwent second look arthroscopy, which showed improved or maintained cartilage. They also reported improved Knee Injury and Osteoarthritis Outcome Scores, Visual Analog Scale pain scores, and Lysholm scores at the 2-year follow-up.[47] Jo and colleagues[48] examined 18 patients with knee OA and found decreased cartilage defect size, improved knee function, and decreased pain after injection of adipose-derived MSCs.

Osteonecrosis of the femoral head

The quality of outcome studies on stem cell therapy for osteonecrosis is improving. Gangji and colleagues[49] showed a reduction in mean volume of femoral necrotic lesions after BMC injection compared with standard care alone at 24 months. A 5-year follow-up study showed patients with early femoral head osteonecrosis were less likely to deteriorate to fractural stage if injected with BMC. Those patients also had a longer survivorship compared with control subjects (52.2 months vs 26.5 months).[50] Hernigou and colleagues[51] reported 69% resolution and 50% decreased mean volume in 342 patients with stage 1 or 2 avascular necrosis. Zhao and colleagues[52] found BMC improved Harris

Hip scores and Femoral Head Low Signal Intensity scores compared with core decompression. Mao and colleagues[53] found that, 5 years after BMC injection, 72 out of 78 hips with osteonecrosis of the femoral head achieved a satisfactory clinical result, whereas only 6 of 78 required a total hip arthroplasty.

Nonunion fractures

A recent study examined 86 patients with diabetes with ankle nonunion treated with BMC and compared results with matched subject with diabetes who underwent standard iliac crest autograft. In the BMC-treated group, 82.1% healed with no major complications. Conversely, 62.3% of the standard care group healed; major complications in that group included 5 amputations, 11 instances of osteonecrosis of fracture wound edge, and 17 infections. Overall, the BMC group showed lower morbidity with greater healing rate.[54]

Anterior cruciate ligament injuries

There is also evidence that BMC injection has beneficial effects in anterior cruciate ligament tears. In a case series by Centeno and colleagues,[55] 10 patients with ACL tears with less than 1 cm retraction underwent an intraligamentous injection of BMC under fluoroscopic guidance. Seven of the 10 patients showed improvement with evidence of improved ligament integrity and increased lower extremity functional scores.

Tendinopathy

Among other soft tissue injuries, there is a greater available volume of studies on tendon injury. Pascual-Garrido and colleagues studied eight patients with refractory patellar tendinopathy for 5 years after bone marrow–derived MSC injections. Of the eight patients, seven were completely satisfied. Statistically significant improvement was seen for most clinical scores including the Knee Injury and Osteoarthritis Outcome Scores activity of daily living, symptom, and sport subscores.[56]

Recent evidence is in favor of the efficacy of stem cells to augment surgical repair of rotator cuff tears. Ellera Gomes and colleagues[57] used mononuclear autologous stem cells to augment conventional rotator cuff repair in 14 patients. MRI analysis after a 12-month follow-up period demonstrated tendon integrity in all cases. Hernigou and colleagues[58] examined 90 patients 10 years after routine arthroscopy with or without BMC injection and found substantial improvement in tendon integrity. In the BMC-treated group, 87% of patients had intact rotator cuffs compared with 44% in the control group.

Safety

PRP and MSC are autologous procedures. Because the cells are removed from and replaced into the same patient, there is no risk of a transfusion reaction or other immune-modulated reactions to the substances when they are reinjected. Risk of disease transmission, such as from an allogenic tissue donor, is also not of concern with these autologous procedures. Wakitani and colleagues[59] studied the safety of bone marrow–derived MSCs for treatment of articular cartilage defects. They monitored 41 patients who received 45 bone marrow MSC injections for 5 to 137 months postprocedure and found no occurrences of infection or tumor growth. Feisst and colleagues[60] cited several phase I and II trials assessing the safety of adipose-derived stem cells without any identifiable significant adverse events. There continues to be ongoing trials assessing the safety and efficacy of bone marrow– and adipose-derived MSCs with promising results.

Further Research

Although the evidence for stem cell application has shown some promise, there remains a need for more robust studies. To date, there are only two studies regarding cartilage treatments with MSCs that are prospective, observational cohorts, one case series with histologic markings and one randomized control trial.[61] With the publication of higher quality research, the appropriate application for stem cell therapies in musculoskeletal medicine will be clarified.

Procedures

Bone marrow

The posterior superior iliac spine is the most commonly accessed landmark for bone marrow aspiration (BMA). This is done either manually with axial force applied to an 11-gauge trephine needle or with a manual drill using a smaller gauge needle.[41] Using ultrasound guidance, a linear-array transducer is typically used (a curvilinear-array transducer may be necessary because of patient body habitus) (**Fig. 3**). The posterior superior iliac spine should be identified with the medial aspect of the probe fixed on it while the lateral portion of the probe is swept between the greater trochanter and the anterior superior iliac spine. Within this arc, the aspirate needle is guided in plane from lateral to medial to the ilium, about 1 to 2 cm from the iliac crest surface for marrow entry (**Fig. 4**). It can then be guided cranially for additional sites (within zone 1 as shown in **Fig. 5**).[62]

Although BMA can be done with anatomic landmarks alone, many practitioners prefer some type of image guidance. Often, fluoroscopic guidance is used to identify the optimal entry point. Ultrasound guidance is used to identify thicker areas of bone where marrow can be more efficiently aspirated. If the needle is introduced into a thinner area of bone, it can pass through the bone as it is being advanced and enter the pelvic cavity. The trajectory of the needle is safest when following a course relatively perpendicular to the thicker portion of the ilium; this is enhanced with ultrasound guidance. Furthermore, surrounding structures including the superior cluneal nerve and superior gluteal vessels may be identified with ultrasound to avoid injuring them during the procedure. In addition, given the discomfort associated with this procedure, ultrasound is helpful to increase the success of aspiration on the first attempt, which avoids the need for multiple trials.

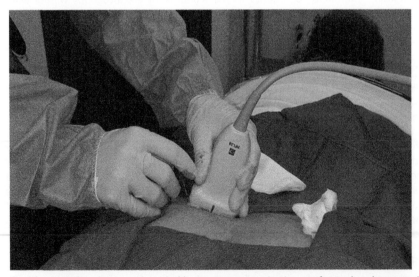

Fig. 3. Approach for ultrasound-guided bone marrow aspiration performed at the posterior superior iliac spine.

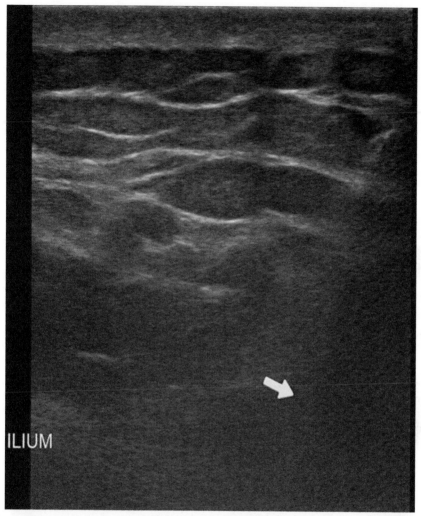

ILIUM

Fig. 4. Ultrasound image of needle (*arrow*) visualized in-plane for bone marrow aspiration.

Discomfort is common after the procedure, but increased donor site pain, discharge, erythema, chills, sweating, or fever should prompt the patient to return for a re-evaluation to inspect the area for infection, hematoma, or other postprocedural complications. Other reported complications following BMA are fracture, sciatic nerve palsy, lateral femoral cutaneous nerve injury, soft tissue injury, and sacroiliac joint injury.[63] Hernigou and colleagues[62] noted only 8 complications in 1800 BMA procedures. Another study noted 410 cadaveric trocar entries (parallel in various sectors) with 114 medial or lateral table breaches (28%).[64]

Adipose
Another viable source for adult MSCs is adipose tissue; however, it is the stromal fractional layer of adipose that contains the MSCs. Lipoaspirate is typically most easily obtained from the gluteal and abdominal regions. Alternative sites include medial or

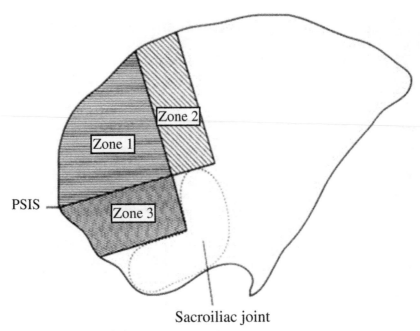

Fig. 5. The regions to initiate needle entry for bone marrow aspiration, with zone 1 preferred and zones 2 and 3 being secondary choices. PSIS, posterior superior iliac spine.

lateral thigh, lateral abdomen, and the greater trochanteric region. Most lipoaspirations can be performed without the need for guidance. Ultrasound is useful to determine the thickness of adipose to choose the optimal position to prepare for the procedure, especially in thinner patients (**Figs. 6** and **7**).[63]

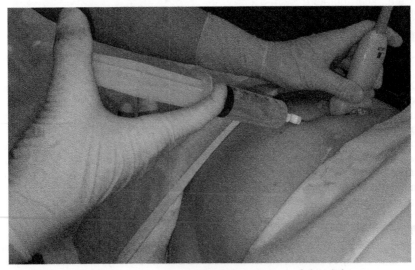

Fig. 6. Approach for ultrasound-guided needle lipoaspiration of the abdomen.

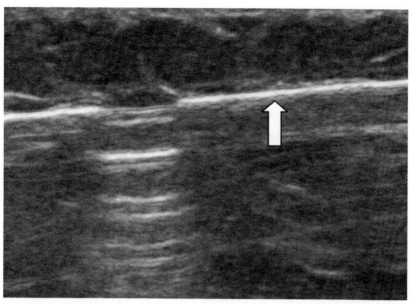

Fig. 7. Ultrasound image with needle (*arrow*) visualized in-plane within subcutaneous adipose tissue for lipoaspiration.

Once the site has been determined, it should be marked and the area should be cleansed with a chlorhexidine-alcohol solution and draped in the usual manner. A solution of 2 mL of 1% lidocaine with epinephrine (to reduce local bleeding) and 8 mL of normal saline solution is made. A lesser degree of anesthetic infiltration maximizes cell viability of the aspirate. The usual goal of a lipoaspiration for orthopedic conditions is 12 to 20 mL of liquefied adipose.[63]

With the advent of the microcannula, cell-friendly equipment, and low-volume techniques, fewer complications occur. This procedure harvests a relatively low volume of aspirate, and therefore skin dimpling is uncommon. Maione and colleagues[64] reviewed 1000 cosmetic surgery cases for postprocedure complications with a mean aspiration volume of 68 mL, which is significantly greater than that proposed for the current procedure. There were 85 donor site complications (two hematomas and 83 local deformities) and five recipient site complications (four infections and one graft rupture).

SUMMARY

The current evidence for the treatment of various orthopedic conditions has documented the long-term complications and pitfalls of corticosteroid injections. Orthobiologics offer new treatment options for these conditions by potentiating tissue healing and regeneration. PRP and MSC treatments (bone marrow and adipose derived) have demonstrated efficacy in in vitro and animal and human studies. The best clinical evidence for PRP in the treatment of tendinopathies exists for chronic lateral epicondylosis, but there is also good evidence for PRP in the treatment of various other tendoninopathies and for ulnar collateral ligament of the elbow injuries. There is also evidence for PRP in the treatment of knee OA, with benefits lasting 9 to 12 months. There is evolving evidence for the role of MSCs in the treatment of various cartilage conditions including OA, including various animal models and human case studies and case series. Ongoing and future research will continue to illuminate the most appropriate and effective applications of these emerging therapies. Ultrasound is helpful in assisting in venipuncture in difficult cases, and in assisting in the harvest of bone marrow and adipose tissue. Most importantly, ultrasound serves to provide guidance for the precise delivery of these biologic agents into the targeted joint, tendon, or ligament.

REFERENCES

1. Coombes BK, Bisset L, Vicenzino B. Efficacy and safety of corticosteroid injections and other injections for management of tendinopathy: a systematic review of randomized controlled trials. Lancet 2010;376:1751–67.
2. Coombes BK, Bisset L, Brooks P, et al. Effect of corticosteroid injection, physiotherapy, or both on clinical outcomes in patients with unilateral lateral epicondalgia: a randomized controlled trial. JAMA 2013;309(5):461–9.
3. Grambart ST. Sports medicine and platelet-rich plasma: nonsurgical therapy. Clin Podiatr Med Surg 2015;32(1):99–107.
4. Okuda K, Kawase T, Momose M, et al. Platelet-rich plasma contains high levels of platelet-derived growth factor and transforming growth factor-beta and modulates the proliferation of periodontally related cells in vitro. J Periodontol 2003; 74(6):849–57.
5. Nguyen RT, Borstein J, McInnis K. Applications of platelet-rich plasma in musculoskeletal and sports medicine: an evidence-based approach. PM R 2011;3: 226–50.
6. Khan M, Bedi A. Cochrane in CORR ®: platelet-rich therapies for musculoskeletal soft tissue injuries. Clin Orthop Relat Res 2015;473(7):2207–13.
7. Mishra A, Harmon K, Woodall J, et al. Sports medicine applications of platelet rich plasma. Curr Pharm Biotechnol 2012;13:1185–95.
8. Dohan Ehrenfest DM, Rasmusson L, Albrektsson T. Classification of platelet concentrates, from pure platelet-rich plasma (PPRP) to leucocyte- and platelet-rich fibrin (L-PRF). Trends Biotechnol 2009;27:158–67.
9. Dohan Ehrenfest DM, Bielecki T, Mishra A, et al. In search of a consensus terminology in the field of platelet concentrates for surgical use: platelet-rich plasma (PRP), platelet-rich fibrin (PRF), fibrin glue polymerization and leukocytes. Curr Pharm Biotechnol 2012;13:1131–7.
10. DeLong JM, Russell RP, Mazzocca AD. Platelet-rich plasma: the PAW classification system. Arthroscopy 2012;28:998–1009.
11. Mautner K, Malanga GA, Smith J, et al. A call for a standard classification system for future biologic research: the rationale for new PRP nomenclature. PM R 2015; 7(4 Suppl):S53–9.
12. Kajikawa Y, Morihara T, Sakamoto H, et al. Platelet-rich plasma enhances the initial mobilization of circulation-derived cells for tendon healing. J Cell Physiol 2008;215(3):837–45.
13. McCarrel TM, Mall NA, Lee AS, et al. Considerations for the use of platelet-rich plasma in orthopedics. Sports Med 2014;44(8):1025–36.
14. Reusz G, Csomos A. The role of ultrasound guidance for vascular access. Curr Opin Anaesthesiol 2015;28(6):710–6.
15. Mazzocca AD, McCarthy MB, Chowaniec DM, et al. Platelet-rich plasma differs according to preparation method and human variability. J Bone Joint Surg Am 2012;94(4):308–16.

16. Malanga G, Nakamura R. The role of regenerative medicine in the treatment of sports injuries. Phys Med Rehabil Clin N Am 2014;25(4):881–95.
17. Giannini S, Buda R, Vannini F, et al. One-step bone marrow-derived cell transplantation in talar osteochondral lesions. Clin Orthop Relat Res 2009;467: 3307–20.
18. Hernigou P, Beaujean F. Treatment of osteonecrosis with autologous bone marrow grafting. Clin Orthop Relat Res 2002;405:14–23.
19. Centeno CJ, Busse D, Kisiday J, et al. Regeneration of meniscus cartilage in a knee treated with percutaneously implanted autologous mesenchymal stem cells. Med Hypotheses 2008;71:900–8.
20. Centeno CJ, Busse D, Kisiday J, et al. Increased knee cartilage volume in degenerative joint disease using percutaneously implanted, autologous mesenchymal stem cells. Pain Physician 2008;11:343–53.
21. Centeno CJ, Kisiday J, Freeman M, et al. Partial regeneration of the human hip via autologous bone marrow nucleated cell transfer: a case study. Pain Physician 2006;9:253–6.
22. Wakitani S, Nawata M, Tensho K, et al. Repair of articular cartilage defects in the patello-femoral joint with autologous bone marrow mesenchymal cell transplantation: three case reports involving nine defects in five knees. J Tissue Eng Regen Med 2007;1:74–9.
23. Pak J. Regeneration of human bones in hip osteonecrosis and human cartilage in knee osteoarthritis with autologous adipose tissue-derived stem cells: a case series. J Med Case Rep 2011;5:296.
24. Nejadnik H, Hui JH, Choong EP, et al. Autologous bone marrow-derived mesenchymal stem cells versus autologous chondrocyte implantation: an observational cohort study. Am J Sports Med 2010;38:1110–6.
25. Caplan AI. All MSCs are pericytes? Cell Stem Cell 2008;3(3):229–30.
26. Dominici M, Le Blanc K, Mueller I, et al. Minimal criteria for defining multipotent mesenchymal stromal cells. The International Society for Cellular Therapy position statement. Cytotherapy 2006;8(4):315–7.
27. Aggarwal S, Pittenger MF. Human mesenchymal stem cells modulate allogeneic immune cell responses. Transplantation 2005;105:1815–22.
28. Iyer S, Rojas M. Anti-inflammatory effects of mesenchymal stem cells: novel concept for future therapies. Expert Opin Biol Ther 2008;8:569–82.
29. Uccelli A, Moretta L, Pistoia V. Mesenchymal stem cells in health and disease. Nat Rev Immunol 2008;8:726–36.
30. Weiss DJ, Bertoncello I, Borok Z, et al. Stem cells and cell therapies in lung biology and lung diseases. Proc Am Thorac Soc 2011;8:223–72.
31. Yagi H, Soto-Gutierrez A, Kitagawa Y. Bone marrow mesenchymal stromal cells attenuate organ injury induced by LPS and burn. Cell Transplant 2010;19:823–30.
32. Guan XJ, Song L, Han FF, et al. Mesenchymal stem cells protect cigarette smoke-damaged lung and pulmonary function partly via VEGF-VEGF receptors. J Cell Biochem 2013;114:323–35.
33. Spaggiari GM, Abdelrazik H, Becchetti F, et al. MSCs inhibit monocyte-derived DC maturation and function by selectively interfering with the generation of immature DCs: central role of MSC-derived prostaglandin E2. Blood 2009;113: 6576–83.
34. Selmani Z, Naji A, Zidi I, et al. Human leukocyte antigen-G5 secretion by human mesenchymal stem cells is required to suppress T lymphocyte and natural killer function and to induce CD4+CD25highFOXP3+regulatory T cells. Stem Cells 2008;26:212–22.

35. Ren G, Zhang L, Zhao X, et al. Mesenchymal stem cell-mediated immunosuppression occurs via concerted action of chemokines and nitric oxide. Cell Stem Cell 2008;2:141–50.

36. Ezquer F, Ezquer M, Contador D, et al. The antidiabetic effect of mesenchymal stem cells is unrelated to their transdifferentiation potential but to their capability to restore Th1/Th2 balance and to modify the pancreatic microenvironment. Stem Cells 2012;30:1664–74.

37. Tollervey JR, Lunyak VV. Adult stem cells: simply a tool for regenerative medicine or an additional piece in the puzzle of human aging? Cell Cycle 2011;10: 4173–6.

38. Tidball JG, Villalta SA. Regulatory interactions between muscle and the immune system during muscle regeneration. Am J Physiol Regul Integr Comp Physiol 2010;298:R1173–87.

39. Choi EW, Shin IS, Lee HW, et al. Transplantation of CTLA4lg gene-transduced adipose tissue-derived mesenchymal stem cells reduces inflammatory immune response and improves Th1/Th2 balance in experimental autoimmune thyroiditis. J Gene Med 2011;13:3–16.

40. Kong Q, Sun B, Bai S, et al. Administration of bone marrow stromal cells ameliorates experimental autoimmune myasthenia gravis by altering the balance of Th1/Th2/Th17/Treg cell subsets through the secretion of TGF-β. J Neuroimmunol 2009;207:83–91.

41. Berenson JR, Yellin O, Blumenstein B, et al. Using a powered bone marrow biopsy system results in shorter procedures, causes less residual pain to adult patients, and yields larger specimens. Diagn Pathol 2011;6:23.

42. Caplan AI. Review: mesenchymal stem cells: cell-based reconstructive therapy in orthopedics. Tissue Eng 2005;11:1198–211.

43. Goldring MB. The role of the chondrocyte in osteoarthritis. Arthritis Rheum 2000; 43:1916–26.

44. Davatchi F, Abdollahi BS, Mohyeddin M, et al. Mesenchymal stem cell therapy for knee osteoarthritis: preliminary report of four patients. Int J Rheum Dis 2011;14: 211–5.

45. Emadedin M, Aghdami N, Taghiyar L, et al. Intra-articular injection of autologous mesenchymal stem cells in six patients with knee osteoarthritis. Arch Iran Med 2012;15:422–8.

46. Sampson S, Botto-Van Bemden A, Aufiero D. Stem cell therapies for treatment of cartilage and bone disorders: osteoarthritis, avascular necrosis and non-union fractures. PM R 2015;7(4):S26–32.

47. Koh YG, Choi YJ. Infrapatellar fat pad-derived mesenchymal stem cell therapy for knee osteoarthritis. Knee 2012;19:902–7.

48. Jo CH, Lee YG, Shin WH, et al. Intra-articular injection of mesenchymal stem cells for the treatment of osteoarthritis of the knee: a proof-of-concept clinical trial. Stem Cells 2014;32(5):1254–66.

49. Gangji V, Hauzeur JP, Matos C, et al. Treatment of osteonecrosis of the femoral head with implantation of autologous bone-marrow cells: a pilot study. J Bone Joint Surg Am 2004;86(6):1153–60.

50. Gangji V, De Maertelaer V, Hauzeur JP. Autologous bone marrow cell implantation in the treatment of non-traumatic osteonecrosis of the femoral head: five year follow-up of a prospective controlled study. Bone 2011;49(5):1005–9.

51. Hernigou P, Poignard A, Zilber S, et al. Cell therapy of hip osteonecrosis with autologous bone marrow grafting. Indian J Orthop 2009;43(1):40–5.

52. Zhao D, Cui D, Wang B, et al. Treatment of early stage osteonecrosis of the femoral head with autologous implantation of bone marrow-derived and cultured mesenchymal stem cells. Bone 2012;50(1):325–30.

53. Mao Q, Jin H, Liao F, et al. The efficacy of targeted intraarterial delivery of concentrated autologous bone marrow containing mononuclear cells in the treatment of osteonecrosis of the femoral head: a five year follow-up study. Bone 2013;57(2):509–16.

54. Flouzat-Lachaniette CH, Heyberger C, Bouthors C, et al. Osteogenic progenitors in bone marrow aspirates have clinical potential for tibial non-unions healing in diabetic patient. Int Orthop 2015;1–5.

55. Centeno CJ, Pitts J, Al-Sayegh H, et al. Anterior cruciate ligament tears treated with percutaneous injection of autologous bone marrow nucleated cells: a case series. J Pain Res 2015;8:437–47.

56. Pascual-Garrido C, Rolón A, Makino A. Treatment of chronic patellar tendinopathy with autologous bone marrow stem cells: a 5-year-followup. Stem Cells Int 2012;2012:953510.

57. Ellera Gomes JL, da Silva RC, Silla LM, et al. Conventional rotator cuff repair complemented by the aid of mononuclear autologous stem cells. Knee Surg Sports Traumatol Arthrosc 2012;20(2):373–7.

58. Hernigou P, Flouzat Lachaniette CH, Delambre J, et al. Biologic augmentation of rotator cuff repair with mesenchymal stem cells during arthroscopy improves healing and prevents further tears: a case-controlled study. Int Orthop 2014; 38(9):1811–8.

59. Wakitani S, Okabe T, Horibe S, et al. Safety of autologous bone marrow-derived mesenchymal stem cell transplantation for cartilage repair in 41 patients with 45 joints followed for up to 11 years and 5 months. J Tissue Eng Regen Med 2011; 5(2):146–50.

60. Feisst V, Meidinger S, Locke MB. From bench to bedside: use of human adipose-derived stem cells. Stem Cells Cloning 2015;8:149–62.

61. Murrell WD, Anz AW, Badsha H, et al. Regenerative treatments to enhance orthopedic surgical outcome. PM R 2015;7(4):S41–52.

62. Hernigou J, Picard L, Alves A, et al. Understanding bone safety zones during bone marrow aspiration from the iliac crest: the sector rule. Int Orthop 2014;38: 2377–84.

63. Bowen JE. Technical issues in harvesting and concentrating stem cells (bone marrow and adipose). PM R 2015;7(4):S8–15.

64. Maione L, Vinci V, Klinger M, et al. Autologous fat graft by needle: analysis of complications after 1000 patients. Ann Plast Surg 2015;74:277–80.

Advanced Ultrasound-Guided Interventions for Tendinopathy

Evan Peck, MD[a,b,*], Elena Jelsing, MD[c], Kentaro Onishi, DO[d]

KEYWORDS

- High volume • Musculoskeletal • Percutaneous • Tendinosis • Tendon
- Sonography • Tenotomy • Ultrasound

KEY POINTS

- Evolving research has shown that tendinopathy is primarily a degenerative condition within the tendon, termed angiofibroblastic hyperplasia, with a likely secondary neurogenic inflammatory component outside the tendon in the surrounding milieu, and this pathophysiologic understanding is reflected in novel percutaneous treatment approaches.
- Ultrasound is an important imaging tool for diagnosis of tendon disorders and for image-guided interventions.
- Percutaneous needle tenotomy, percutaneous ultrasonic tenotomy, high-volume injection, and percutaneous needle scraping are promising new treatments for tendinopathy, but further research is needed with larger, high-quality, randomized controlled trials to further define their efficacy and role.

INTRODUCTION

Tendinopathy is an important cause of musculoskeletal pain and disability. Although traditionally thought to be an inflammatory condition and described as tendonitis, subsequent data showed it to be primarily a degenerative problem, more appropriately labeled tendinosis.[1–3] Tendinosis occurs with multiple microtrauma, leading to degeneration of tenocytes and the extracellular matrix, which fail to mature or remodel into

Disclosures: The authors have no disclosures.
[a] Section of Sports Health, Department of Orthopaedic Surgery, Cleveland Clinic Florida, 525 Okeechobee Boulevard, Suite 1400, West Palm Beach, FL 33401, USA; [b] Charles E. Schmidt College of Medicine, Florida Atlantic University, Boca Raton, FL 33431, USA; [c] Department of Physical Medicine and Rehabilitation, Mayo Clinic College of Medicine, Mayo Clinic Sports Medicine Center, Minneapolis, MN 55403, USA; [d] Department of Physical Medicine and Rehabilitation, University of Pittsburgh Medical Center, Pittsburgh, PA 15213, USA
* Corresponding author. Section of Sports Health, Department of Orthopaedic Surgery, Cleveland Clinic Florida, 525 Okeechobee Boulevard, Suite 1400, West Palm Beach, FL 33401.
E-mail address: pecke@ccf.org

Phys Med Rehabil Clin N Am 27 (2016) 733–748
http://dx.doi.org/10.1016/j.pmr.2016.04.008
1047-9651/16/$ – see front matter © 2016 Elsevier Inc. All rights reserved.

normal tendon.[4] This process has been described as angiofibroblastic hyperplasia, consisting of fibroblasts, vascular hyperplasia, and disorganized collagen.[3,4] Risk factors for the development of tendinopathy include ballistic performance, repeated or high-force eccentric contractions, an adjacent convex surface or apex of a concavity, muscles that cross 2 joints, scant vascular supply, and repetitive tension.[3,4]

Although inflammatory cells are generally not seen within the tendon substance in tendinopathy, inflammatory mediators have been found in the tendon's surrounding milieu, suggesting that tendinopathy is not solely degenerative.[5] This condition has been described as neurogenic inflammation, consisting of inflammatory mediators that induce matrix metalloproteinase production, leading to degradation of the extracellular matrix of the tendon and promoting neoangiogenesis.[5,6] These abnormal neovessels are associated with neonerves, theorized to contribute to the pain of tendinopathy.[6]

Tendinopathy has historically been treated with a wide range of interventions,[7] including rest; cryotherapy; therapeutic ultrasound (US); stretching; strengthening, including eccentric-biased strengthening; taping; bracing; oral and topical analgesics and nonsteroidal antiinflammatory drugs (NSAIDs); extracorporeal shock-wave therapy; topical vasodilators; and corticosteroid injections.[8,9] Few of these treatments have been shown to be effective, and corticosteroid injections, once a mainstay of tendinopathy treatment, have been found to be harmful to tendons.[10] Consequently, clinicians have sought safer and more effective interventions for the treatment of this condition.

With the emergence of diagnostic musculoskeletal US, clinicians are better able to evaluate tendinopathy at the point of care while using an easily portable, safe, cost-effective, and high-resolution imaging modality. US is able to characterize tendon disorders in detail by assessing the tendon's fibrillar architecture; identifying tears, enthesophytes, cortical irregularity, and intrasubstance calcifications; and quantifying hyperemia.[7] With the use of US, the specific location of a disorder within a tendon can be more accurately and completely delineated. As the diagnostic capability of musculoskeletal US has improved, clinicians have also developed more advanced interventional procedures facilitated by US guidance, with procedural mechanisms corresponding with the improved understanding of tendon disorders outlined earlier. These procedures include percutaneous needle tenotomy (PNT), percutaneous ultrasonic tenotomy (PUT), high-volume injection (HVI), percutaneous needle scraping (PNS), and orthobiologic interventions. This article reviews common percutaneous US-guided procedures for the treatment of tendinopathy using chiefly some form of mechanical debridement or similar intervention to stimulate regeneration. For a discussion of orthobiologic substances, such as platelet-rich plasma and mesenchymal stem cells, see Malanga G, Abdelshahed D, Jayaram P: Orthobiologic Interventions Utilizing Ultrasound Guidance, in this issue.

PERCUTANEOUS NEEDLE TENOTOMY

US-guided PNT has been used as an independent treatment strategy as well as being combined with orthobiologic products. PNT involves repeatedly passing a needle through a tendon with the goal of disrupting the chronic degenerative process, including scar tissue, and encouraging localized bleeding and fibroblast proliferation, which can lead to growth factor release, collagen formation, and ultimately healing.[9,11]

There is minimal research on the outcomes of US-guided PNT alone. Some of the first published studies that described PNT also involved the injection of local anesthetic and corticosteroid. In 2006, McShane and colleagues[8] reported the results of

55 US-guided elbow common extensor tendon PNTs followed by infiltration of a mixture of corticosteroid and bupivacaine. Following this procedure, 80% of participants reported excellent or good outcomes, with no adverse events among any of the subjects, at an average follow-up of 28 months. In 2008, McShane and colleagues[12] published a similar study of PNT for elbow common extensor tendinosis, but corticosteroid injection was not used in conjunction with the procedure. Of the 52 patients who participated in the study, 92% reported excellent or good outcomes at an average follow-up of 22 months, suggesting that omitting corticosteroid from the procedure improved clinical outcomes.

These findings were similar to a study published by Zhu and colleagues,[13] which also reported 87% excellent or good outcomes after a US-guided elbow common extensor tendon PNT plus corticosteroid and local anesthetic injection, although some patients were treated with this intervention multiple times at intervals of 1 to 2 weeks. Note that, since these studies were published, newer evidence has been published suggesting that injecting corticosteroid directly into a tendon may be harmful and thus should generally be avoided.[10]

In 2010, Housner and colleagues[14] reported similar results with US-guided patellar tendon PNT. Of 47 subjects who underwent the procedure, 72% returned to activity with no or only minimal pain, 81% reported excellent or good satisfaction scores, and only 1 tendon ruptured, at 6 weeks postprocedure. Housner and colleagues[11] also reported the prospective outcomes of US-guided PNT performed on 5 patellar tendons, 4 Achilles tendons, 1 proximal gluteus medius tendon, 1 proximal iliotibial band, 1 proximal hamstring tendon, 1 elbow common extensor tendon, and 1 proximal rectus femoris tendon. In all of these patients, visual analog scale (VAS) scores were significantly lower at the 4-week and 12-week follow-up periods and there were no reported complications. Similarly, Jacobson and colleagues[15] published their retrospective results following US-guided PNT on 11 gluteus medius tendons, 2 gluteus minimus tendons, 8 hamstring tendons, and 1 tensor fascia lata tendon. Of these patients, 45% reported marked improvement, 37% reported some improvement, 9% reported no change, and 9% reported worsening symptoms. There is also 1 published case report of clinical and sonographic improvement after US-guided PNT of the supraspinatus tendon.[16]

Some investigations have used US-guided PNT as the control group in studies comparing this intervention with PNT plus the addition of an orthobiologic product. Krey and colleagues[9] identified 2 studies involving US-guided PNT in a systematic literature review. The first, conducted by Rha and colleagues,[17] showed significant subjective clinical improvements at 6 months following US-guided PNT of the supraspinatus tendon. In this study, PNT alone was compared with PNT plus platelet-rich plasma injections. Similarly, Stenhouse and colleagues[18] compared US-guided common extensor tendon PNT alone versus PNT plus autologous conditioned plasma injections. Following PNT alone, subjective symptom scales significantly improved at both 2 and 6 months postprocedure. Of note, in both of these studies, PNT was performed twice, at 1 month apart. Mishra and colleagues[19] subsequently published a randomized controlled trial comparing PNT alone versus PNT with platelet-rich plasma injection for the treatment of elbow common extensor tendinopathy in 230 patients. In the PNT alone group, pain scores improved 56% versus baseline and treatment success was 68% at 24 weeks postprocedure.

In summary, there has only been 1 prospective study of the outcomes of US-guided PNT as the sole intervention for tendinopathy.[11] However, all of the present PNT literature consistently notes improvement in symptoms and reports rare complications. Larger, randomized controlled trials are needed. Further prospective research is also needed to determine whether PNT should be repeated when a patient experiences suboptimal results or partial improvement and if so, when this is indicated. In addition, future investigations should address whether patients with partial-thickness tears fare better or worse than those with tendinopathy alone when treated with PNT.

SAMPLE PROCEDURE: PERCUTANEOUS NEEDLE TENOTOMY OF THE ELBOW COMMON EXTENSOR TENDON

The patient is placed in a supine position with the elbow flexed to 60° and the pronated forearm resting comfortably on the patient's abdomen. The proximal end of a high-frequency (>10 MHz) linear-array US transducer is then placed over the palpable bony prominence of the lateral epicondyle (**Fig. 1**). With the acoustic landmarks of the lateral epicondyle and the radial head visible, a long-axis view of the common extensor tendon is obtained (**Fig. 2**). The area of tendinopathy is identified sonographically, typically characterized by tendon thickening; loss of normal fibrillar echotexture; hypoechogenicity; hyperemia, as visualized with color or power Doppler imaging; and possibly partial-thickness tears, represented by anechoic tendon defects that may be more conspicuous with transducer compression. The authors generally do not recommend that full-thickness tendon tears are treated with PNT, based on the available literature and proposed mechanism of action.

The procedural site and surrounding area is then prepared and draped in a sterile fashion, and the transducer is covered using a sterile transducer cover kit. Then, a 25-gauge needle is used under direct sonographic guidance to anesthetize the skin, subcutaneous tissue, and tendon with a rapid-onset local anesthetic, such as lidocaine. This needle is removed. Thereafter, under direct sonographic visualization,

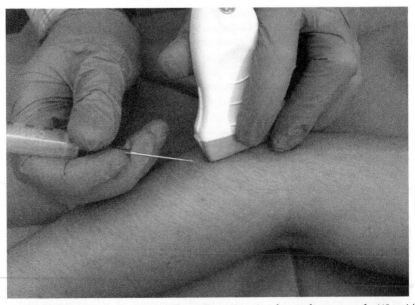

Fig. 1. Patient, clinician, transducer, and needle positioning for performance of a US-guided percutaneous needle tenotomy of the elbow common extensor tendon. Sterile transducer cover not shown. Left, distal; right, proximal.

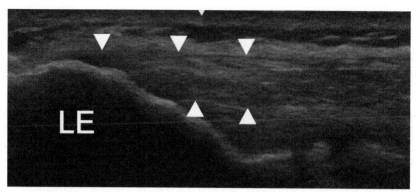

Fig. 2. US image of elbow common extensor tendinopathy shown long axis to the transducer. Note thickening, hypoechogenicity, and loss of normal fibrillar echotexture of the tendon. Arrowheads indicate superficial and deep borders of the common extensor tendon. Bottom, deep; left, proximal; right, distal; top, superficial. LE, lateral epicondyle.

using a distal-to-proximal, needle-in-plane approach, a 19-gauge needle is inserted into the same entry site as the prior needle, and the tip is guided into the area of tendinopathy (**Fig. 3**). The US transducer and needle are parallel to the fibers of the tendon in this view. With continuous sonographic visualization, the needle tip is then repeatedly passed through the tendinopathic area until the tendon has been adequately fenestrated. Adequate fenestration is subjective but is often appreciated by markedly less resistance perceived when the needle traverses the tendon. Care must be taken to not pass the needle deeper than approximately 50% of the total footprint of the lateral epicondyle in order to avoid inadvertent piercing of the radial collateral ligament, which lies deep to the common extensor tendon.[20]

It is recommended that additional local anesthetic, such as lidocaine or ropivacaine, is kept in a syringe attached to the tenotomy needle throughout the procedure, so that additional local anesthetic may be administered if the patient experiences discomfort. However, although patient comfort should be respected, local anesthetic use should

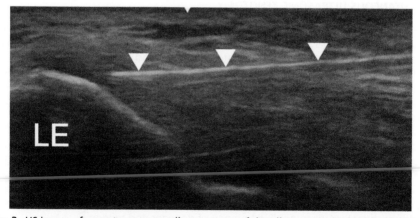

Fig. 3. US image of percutaneous needle tenotomy of the elbow common extensor tendon, with both tendon and needle shown long axis to the transducer. Arrowheads indicate the needle. Bottom, deep; left, proximal; right, distal; top, superficial. LE, lateral epicondyle.

otherwise be judicious, because all local anesthetics may be toxic to tenocytes.[21] Among these, bupivacaine may be the most toxic to tenocytes and its use during tendon procedures is generally not recommended by the authors.[22]

The transducer should be periodically rotated 90° during the procedure to obtain a short-axis view of the common extensor tendon to ensure that the entire area of tendinopathy is being treated. In the long-axis view, the needle can also be used to abrade the cortex of the lateral epicondyle and any enthesophytes, potentially stimulating additional tendon healing. Intrasubstance tendon calcifications may also be disrupted by the needle. Following the procedure, the needle is removed from the skin, pressure is applied to the area to achieve adequate hemostasis, and a sterile adhesive dressing is placed over the procedural site.

There are many variables to this procedure, such as the size of the needle used for the tenotomy and the number of passes with the needle. Needles ranging from 16 to 22 gauge have been described in the literature.[11,13,15] The number of needle passes may vary based on numerous factors, such as patient characteristics, severity and size of the tendinopathic area, presence or absence of tears, operator experience and comfort level, and needle gauge used. The number of needle passes ranges from 20 to 40 when it has been specifically noted in the available PNT literature, although the authors have frequently found that up to double this number may be necessary to achieve adequate fenestration and a satisfactory clinical outcome.[14,15]

In addition, there is considerable variability in postprocedural care, such as the avoidance of antiinflammatory medications, the use of bracing, rehabilitation protocols, and return-to-activity guidelines. In general, the authors recommend that the patient remain in a sling for 2 days postprocedure, avoid repeated gripping or heavy lifting activities by the treated limb for 2 weeks postprocedure, perform only active range-of-motion exercises for the first 2 weeks postprocedure with no strengthening or stretching during this 2-week period, and engages in a rehabilitation program and return-to-activity schedule similar to that published by Finnoff and colleagues,[23] culminating in a return to full activities at approximately 8 to 12 weeks postprocedure. In addition, the authors recommend avoidance of NSAIDs for 1 week before the procedure and for 2 weeks following it, at minimum, to avoid suppression of the beneficial and normal inflammatory phase of tendon healing induced by the procedure.

PERCUTANEOUS ULTRASONIC TENOTOMY

US-guided PUT is an evolving procedure for the treatment of recalcitrant tendinopathy. It is currently US Food and Drug Administration approved for elbow common extensor, elbow common flexor/pronator, patellar, and Achilles tendinopathy, as well as plantar fasciopathy. This procedure was inspired by technology derived from the phacoemulsification procedure used during cataract surgery, in which an ultrasonic vibrating tip emulsifies and suctions the internal lens of the eye.[24] In musculoskeletal medicine, the emulsification and debridement process is targeted to angiofibroblastic tissues seen within tendinopathy or fasciopathy under sonographic guidance, and requires a special device that allows debridement and suctioning. The presently available system using this technology consists of a suction and irrigation system connected to a handheld instrument with an ultrasonic vibrating double-lumen needle, which is approximately the size of a conventional 32-mm 18-gauge needle. Based on an animal histologic study, the PUT procedure promotes normal tendon architecture when applied to areas of degenerated tendon.[25]

There are presently 4 published clinical studies of PUT, all case series, and these are summarized in **Table 1**. A total of 67 cases of common extensor, common

Table 1
Clinical studies of PUT

Author(s), Year	Diagnosis Treated	Average Duration of Symptoms (mo)	Sample Size	Outcome Measurements	Results
Elattrache & Morrey,[26] 2013	Patellar tendinopathy	Not reported	16	Return to previous level of play	Approximately 63% of subjects returned to previous level, with >93% verbalizing some improvement.
Koh et al,[27] 2013	Common extensor tendinopathy	13	20	VAS, DASH, sonographic appearance of tendon, patient satisfaction, complications	VAS improvement at week 1, with progressive improvement over 12 mo. DASH improved at 3, 6, and 12 mo postprocedure. At least 85% of tendons showed improved morphologic characteristics at 6 mo postprocedure; 95% of patients verbalized satisfaction.
Barnes et al,[28] 2015	Common extensor and common flexor/pronator tendinopathy	At least 6	12 (CET); 7 (CFPT)	VAS, QuickDASH, MEPS, complications	VAS improvement at week 6, with progressive improvement over 12 mo. QuickDASH and MEPS stayed improved for 12 mo.
Patel,[29] 2015	Plantar fasciopathy	19	12	AOFAS	Average AOFAS improved from 30 to 88. All subjects were pain-free by 24 mo.

All studies noted are case series.
Abbreviations: AOFAS, American Orthopaedic Foot and Ankle Society Ankle-Hindfoot Scale; CET, elbow common extensor tendinopathy; CFPT, elbow common flexor/pronator tendinopathy; DASH, Disabilities of the Arm, Shoulder, and Hand Score; MEPS, Mayo Elbow Performance Score; QuickDASH, shortened version of DASH score.

flexor/pronator, and patellar tendinopathy, as well as plantar fasciopathy, have cumulatively been reported in these studies.[26–29] Improvement in pain and functional scores were noted as early as 1 week[27] and as late as 2 months[29] postprocedure, with no reported complications.

Because these studies are all case series, the relative efficacy of PUT compared with other interventions is currently unknown, and further investigation with prospective randomized controlled trials is needed. In addition, an inherent limitation of case series is the lack of a control group, so spontaneous improvement without PUT cannot be excluded. In addition, it is unclear whether PUT is more cost-effective than other nonsurgical and surgical interventions for tendinopathy, and this also warrants further study.

SAMPLE PROCEDURE: PERCUTANEOUS ULTRASONIC TENOTOMY OF THE PATELLAR TENDON

The patient is placed on an examination table supine with a pillow under the affected knee to support flexion of approximately 45°. As with the PNT procedure, the patient's patellar tendon is then sonographically evaluated to identify the area of tendinopathy and plan the procedure. A surgical marker is used to delineate the device entry point. The device approach can be long axis or short axis to the tendon depending on clinician preference, location of tendinopathy, patient characteristics, and other factors. The long-axis approach is described for this sample procedure. Once the entry point is marked, the patient is draped and prepared in a sterile fashion and the transducer is covered with a sterile transducer cover kit.

Under direct sonographic guidance, a rapid-onset local anesthetic is then administered using a 25-gauge needle to anesthetize the skin, subcutaneous tissue, and patellar tendon. A #11 blade scalpel is then used to make a stab incision to create an entry site for the PUT device, which has a blunt tip. If possible, the stab incision should be passed to the level of the tendon. In addition, the PUT device is advanced under sonographic guidance into the area of tendinopathy within the patellar tendon, where it is activated using a foot pedal (**Figs. 4** and **5**). Frequently, the PUT device needs to be redirected to cover the entire area of tendinopathy, similar to PNT. Following completion of the procedure, wound closure is accomplished using sterile adhesive dressing.

As with PNT, clinical experience and the published literature offer varying recommendations regarding postprocedural activity progression and rehabilitation. The authors recommend that the patient is toe-touch weight bearing on the treated limb using a knee immobilizer and crutches for 1 week, followed by 1 week of 50% partial weight bearing. The patient is instructed to perform knee active range-of-motion exercises starting at 2 days postprocedure and continue for the first 2 weeks postprocedure. The authors also recommend the patient avoid NSAIDs on a similar schedule to that described with the PNT procedure earlier. Because no presently published clinical PUT study has outlined a detailed postprocedural rehabilitation program, the authors generally recommend that subsequent rehabilitation is based on Finnoff and colleagues'[23] guidelines for PNT, with adjustments made as indicated on an individual basis. It is not clear at this time whether a more aggressive or conservative rehabilitation program is warranted for PUT versus PNT, so clinicians should closely follow the course of each patient to appropriately modify rehabilitation and activity progression.

HIGH-VOLUME INJECTION

The interventions described previously in this article focus chiefly on treating the tendon substance, using mechanical debridement to disrupt the angiofibroblastic

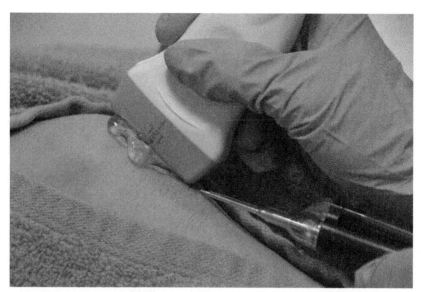

Fig. 4. Patient, clinician, transducer, and instrument positioning for performance of a US-guided PUT of the patellar tendon. Sterile transducer cover not shown. Left, proximal; right, distal.

hyperplasia that is characteristic of tendinosis and to stimulate healing and regeneration of the tendon. In contrast, HVI with respect to tendinopathy treatment focuses on using high volumes of injectate to disrupt neovessels and neonerves, which may diminish neurogenic inflammation, decrease tendon pain, and promote healing. This technique has chiefly been studied in patellar and Achilles tendinopathy, wherein most neovessels and neonerves are sonographically observed between the affected tendon and an adjacent fat pad (ie, patellar tendon and Hoffa fat pad; Achilles tendon and Kager fat pad).

US-guided HVI for the treatment of patellar tendinopathy was initially described in 2008 by Crisp and colleagues.[30] Nine patients with patellar tendinopathy refractory

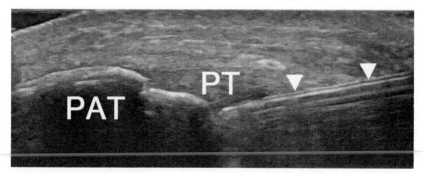

Fig. 5. US image of percutaneous ultrasonic tenotomy of the patellar tendon, with both tendon and tenotomy instrument shown long axis to the transducer. Arrowheads indicate the percutaneous ultrasonic tenotomy instrument. Bottom, deep; left, proximal; right, distal; top, superficial. PAT, patella; PT, patellar tendon. (*Courtesy of* Darryl Barnes, MD, Mayo Clinic Health System, Austin, MN.)

to conservative care with hyperemia noted on power Doppler imaging were treated with a US-guided HVI at the interface between the patellar tendon and Hoffa fat pad. The injection consisted of 10 mL of 0.5% bupivacaine, 25 mg of hydrocortisone, and between 12 and 40 mL of normal saline, determined by the clinician based on the amount of resistance encountered. Compared with baseline values, VAS scores improved significantly at 2 weeks postprocedure, and Victorian Institute of Sport Assessment–Patellar Tendon (VISA-P) scores were improved significantly at 9 months' follow-up.

In 2014, a slightly larger combined retrospective and prospective study of 20 patients with patellar tendinopathy treated with US-guided HVI was reported.[31] A similar technique was used, targeting the patellar tendon–Hoffa fat pad interface, injecting a mixture of 10 mL of 0.5% bupivacaine, 25 mg of hydrocortisone, and 30 mL of normal saline, with no variability of volume based on clinician judgment or amount of resistance. Subjects started an eccentric strengthening rehabilitation program at 4 days postprocedure, nonimpact aerobic exercise at 7 days postprocedure, and returned to sport at 12 days postprocedure at the earliest, depending on individual patient factors and clinical response. At 12 weeks postprocedure, VISA-P scores improved significantly versus baseline, and 38% of subjects returned to full sport participation by that time.

A larger prospective case series was published in 2016, consisting of 44 patients with patellar tendinopathy refractory to conservative care treated with US-guided HVI.[32] Again the interface of the patellar tendon and Hoffa fat pad was the target of treatment, and a mixture of 10 mL of 0.5% bupivacaine, 62,500 IU of aprotinin, and 40 mL of normal saline was used for the injections. At 15 months postprocedure, VAS and VISA-P scores were significantly improved from baseline. Of the 44 subjects, 32 were described by the investigators as physically active, and 72% of these patients returned to sport by 15 months postprocedure at the same level as before symptom onset.

US-guided HVI has also been described for midportion Achilles tendinopathy, and was first reported by Chan and colleagues[33] in 2008. Thirty patients who failed at least 3 months of eccentric strengthening were treated with an HVI consisting of 10 mL of bupivacaine, 25 mg of hydrocortisone, and up to 40 mL of normal saline at the interface between the Achilles tendon and Kager fat pad. Victorian Institute of Sport Assessment–Achilles Tendon (VISA-A) scores significantly improved from baseline at both 4 weeks and 30 weeks postprocedure.

Another case series of 11 patients with recalcitrant midportion Achilles tendinopathy treated with HVI was later reported[34] using a similar technique and an identical injection mixture to Chan and colleagues'[33] study. In this investigation, VISA-A scores significantly improved at 3 weeks postprocedure; there was no long-term follow-up. The investigators also noted significant tendon morphologic changes on US at 3 weeks postprocedure, including significant decreases in neovascularization and tendon thickness. In 2013, Maffulli and colleagues[35] published a larger prospective case series of 94 patients with recalcitrant midportion Achilles tendinopathy treated with an HVI of 10 mL of 0.5% bupivacaine, 25 mg of aprotinin, and up to 40 mL of normal saline. At 12 months postprocedure, VISA-A scores were significantly improved.

In summary, US-guided HVI for the treatment of patellar and midportion Achilles tendinopathy has shown promise in improvement of both pain and functional scores, with positive effects persisting for up to 15 months postprocedure. No complications have been reported for this procedure in any of the published data. Another potential advantage of this procedure is that, because the tendon is not mechanically debrided, rehabilitation and return to activity may progress at a faster rate than with PNT or PUT, although this theory has not been thoroughly investigated. Notably, all of the presently published articles using HVI for tendinopathy treatment are case series; further investigation of this procedure would benefit from randomized controlled trials using a control group or other tendinopathy interventions, such as PNT, PUT, or orthobiologics.

PERCUTANEOUS NEEDLE SCRAPING

The mechanism of action of PNS is thought to be similar to HVI. With PNS, a needle is directed under US guidance into the tendon–fat pad interface, and a scraping technique is used to mechanically disrupt neovessels and accompanying neonerves, which may accomplish a similar effect as HVI. This procedure was first described by Alfredson[36] in 2011 for the treatment of refractory midportion Achilles tendinopathy. This study included 88 tendons in a case series treated with an open surgical scalpel scraping technique, and 37 tendons treated in a randomized study with patients allocated to either an open surgical scalpel or a PNS technique. For the PNS technique, a 14-gauge needle was inserted from either the medial or lateral side of the tendon under US guidance, and used to separate the ventral side of the tendon from the Kager fat pad. Patients were permitted to weight bear immediately, gradually increasing walking over the first week and bicycling during the second week. Rehabilitation was progressed on an individual basis subsequently. One partial Achilles tendon rupture related to a major trauma was reported, although it is not clear whether this patient was in the open surgical or PNS group. At 18 months postprocedure, VAS was significantly decreased from baseline, with 89% of patients satisfied with the procedure. There were no significant differences in outcome between the open surgical scalpel and PNS groups in the randomized arm of the study. Another investigation using an open surgical scalpel scraping technique was subsequently reported, but no other studies have been published using a US-guided PNS technique for midportion Achilles tendinopathy treatment.[37]

Hall and Rajasekaran[38] in 2015 reported a case of recalcitrant patellar tendinopathy successfully treated with PNS using an 18-gauge needle, with the addition of a 20-mL normal saline HVI administered concurrently. At 6 months postprocedure, the patient had fully returned to sport, with improved VAS, VISA-P, and Blazina scale scores.

In summary, limited literature is presently available on the use of PNS for the treatment of tendinopathy, and this interesting technique warrants more thorough investigation with larger, randomized controlled trials.

SAMPLE PROCEDURE: HIGH-VOLUME INJECTION AND PERCUTANEOUS NEEDLE SCRAPING OF THE MIDPORTION ACHILLES TENDON

In clinical practice, the authors have used a hybrid procedure combining HVI and PNS, given their similar theoretic mechanisms of action, similar rehabilitation and return-to-play guidelines given treatment outside of the tendon substance, and ease of coadministration with a single needle entry point. For this sample procedure, treatment of midportion Achilles tendinopathy is described.

The patient is placed in a prone position. The Achilles tendon is sonographically examined to delineate the area of tendinopathy. In particular, the presence of neovascularization on power Doppler imaging is carefully noted preprocedurally (**Fig. 6**). The patient is then prepared and draped in a sterile fashion, and the transducer is prepared with a sterile transducer cover kit. The transducer is placed short axis to the Achilles tendon, and under direct sonographic guidance a 25-gauge needle is introduced laterally to anesthetize the skin, subcutaneous tissue, and interface

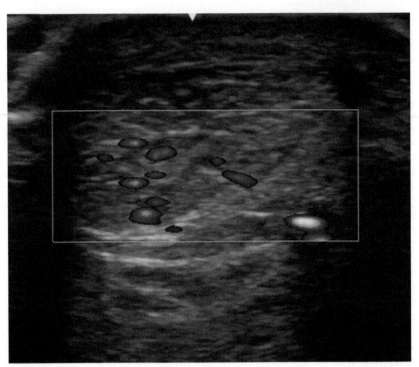

Fig. 6. US image of the Achilles tendon shown in short axis to the transducer, before HVI and PNS procedure. Note power Doppler imaging findings of increased hyperemia, characteristic of abnormal neovessels associated with tendinopathy. Bottom, deep; left, medial; right, lateral; top, superficial.

between the Achilles tendon and Kager fat pad using a rapid-onset local anesthetic such as lidocaine (**Fig. 7**). Care is taken to identify and avoid the nearby sural nerve. Multiple passes while injecting local anesthetic in a more proximal and distal direction along the tendon–fat pad interface are performed, without withdrawing the needle from the skin. The anesthetic needle is subsequently withdrawn and an 18-gauge needle is inserted using the same entry site, using a lateral approach and again taking care to avoid the sural nerve. This needle is used to mechanically separate the ventral surface of the Achilles tendon from the adjacent Kager fat pad, concurrently administering a mixture of 10 mL of 0.5% ropivacaine and 40 mL of normal saline throughout the procedure to assist with tendon–fat pad separation (**Fig. 8**). No corticosteroid is injected because of known deleterious effects of corticosteroid on tendons.[10] Postprocedural scanning often shows diminished neovascularization on power Doppler imaging (**Fig. 9**).

Following the procedure, the patient is allowed to weight bear as tolerated but should not participate in any sports or exercise for 1 week aside from casual walking and active range-of-motion ankle exercises. The patient may begin nonimpact light aerobic exercise, light (<60% 1-repetition maximum) isotonic strengthening without an eccentric bias, and stretching in the second postprocedural week. At 2 weeks postprocedure, the patient may begin returning to normal sports and activities depending on individual clinical response.

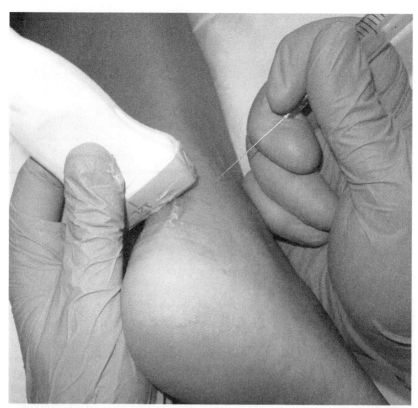

Fig. 7. Patient, clinician, transducer, and needle positioning for performance of a US-guided HVI and PNS procedure of the Achilles tendon. Sterile transducer cover not shown. Left, medial; right, lateral.

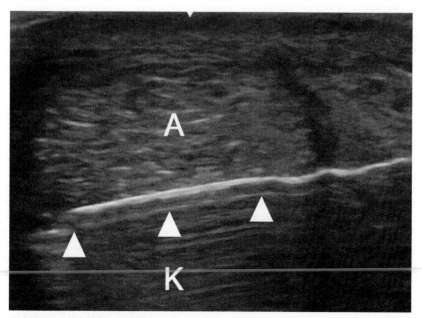

Fig. 8. US image of HVI and PNS procedure of the Achilles tendon, with tendon shown short axis and needle shown long axis to the transducer. Arrowheads indicate the needle. Bottom, deep; left, medial; right, lateral; top, superficial. A, Achilles tendon; K, Kager fat pad.

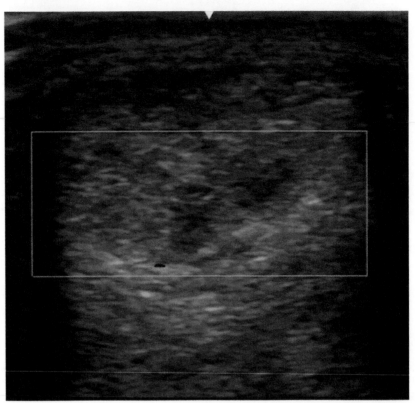

Fig. 9. US image of the Achilles tendon shown short axis to the transducer, immediately following HVI and PNS procedure performed on the tendon shown in **Fig. 6**. Note power Doppler imaging findings of markedly decreased hyperemia versus preprocedural image, suggestive of diminished neovessels as a result of the procedure. Bottom, deep; left, medial; right, lateral; top, superficial.

SUMMARY

The improved understanding of tendinopathy as primarily a degenerative condition, with a likely secondary neurogenic inflammatory component, has promoted the development of novel treatments focused on this pathophysiology. The significant advancements in the use of musculoskeletal US for diagnostic and interventional purposes have played a critical role in the development of these interventions. Based on present data, PNT, PUT, HVI, and PNS seem to be safe, and efficacy shows early promise. However, current studies regarding these interventions are of limited size and evidence quality. Further research should focus on these treatments in larger randomized controlled trials, perhaps compared with or in conjunction with orthobiologic injections, to further define their safety, efficacy, cost-effectiveness, and role in the treatment of this important and challenging clinical problem in musculoskeletal medicine.

REFERENCES

1. Astrom M, Rausing A. Chronic Achilles tendinopathy. A survey of surgical and histopathologic findings. Clin Orthop Relat Res 1995;316:151–64.

2. Khan KM, Cook JL, Bonar F, et al. Histopathology of common tendinopathies. Update and implications for clinical management. Sports Med 1999;27(6):393–408.
3. Khan KM, Cook JL, Taunton JE, et al. Overuse tendinosis, not tendinitis part 1: a new paradigm for a difficult clinical problem. Phys Sportsmed 2000;28(5):38–48.
4. Kraushaar BS, Nirschl RP. Tendinosis of the elbow (tennis elbow). Clinical features and findings of histological, immunohistochemical, and electron microscopy studies. J Bone Joint Surg Am 1999;81(2):259–78.
5. Abate M, Silbernagel KG, Siljeholm C, et al. Pathogenesis of tendinopathies: inflammation or degeneration? Arthritis Res Ther 2009;11(3):235.
6. Dakin SG, Dudhia J, Smith RK. Resolving an inflammatory concept: the importance of inflammation and resolution in tendinopathy. Vet Immunol Immunopathol 2014;158(3–4):121–7.
7. Chiavaras MM, Jacobson JA. Ultrasound-guided tendon fenestration. Semin Musculoskelet Radiol 2013;17(1):85–90.
8. McShane JM, Nazarian LN, Harwood MI. Sonographically guided percutaneous needle tenotomy for treatment of common extensor tendinosis in the elbow. J Ultrasound Med 2006;25(10):1281–9.
9. Krey D, Borchers J, McCamey K. Tendon needling for treatment of tendinopathy: a systematic review. Phys Sportsmed 2015;43(1):80–6.
10. Coombes BK, Bisset L, Brooks P, et al. Effect of corticosteroid injection, physiotherapy, or both on clinical outcomes in patients with unilateral lateral epicondylalgia: a randomized controlled trial. JAMA 2013;309(5):461–9.
11. Housner JA, Jacobson JA, Misko R. Sonographically guided percutaneous needle tenotomy for the treatment of chronic tendinosis. J Ultrasound Med 2009; 28(9):1187–92.
12. McShane JM, Shah VN, Nazarian LN. Sonographically guided percutaneous needle tenotomy for treatment of common extensor tendinosis in the elbow: is a corticosteroid necessary? J Ultrasound Med 2008;27(8):1137–44.
13. Zhu J, Hu B, Xing C, et al. Ultrasound-guided, minimally invasive, percutaneous needle puncture treatment for tennis elbow. Adv Ther 2008;25(10):1031–6.
14. Housner JA, Jacobson JA, Morag Y, et al. Should ultrasound-guided needle fenestration be considered as a treatment option for recalcitrant patellar tendinopathy? A retrospective study of 47 cases. Clin J Sport Med 2010;20(6):488–90.
15. Jacobson JA, Rubin J, Yablon CM, et al. Ultrasound-guided fenestration of tendons about the hip and pelvis: clinical outcomes. J Ultrasound Med 2015; 34(11):2029–35.
16. Settergren R. Treatment of supraspinatus tendinopathy with ultrasound guided dry needling. J Chiropr Med 2013;12(1):26–9.
17. Rha DW, Park GY, Kim YK, et al. Comparison of the therapeutic effects of ultrasound-guided platelet-rich plasma injection and dry needling in rotator cuff disease: a randomized controlled trial. Clin Rehabil 2013;27(2):113–22.
18. Stenhouse G, Sookur P, Watson M. Do blood growth factors offer additional benefit in refractory lateral epicondylitis? A prospective, randomized pilot trial of dry needling as a stand-alone procedure versus dry needling and autologous conditioned plasma. Skeletal Radiol 2013;42(11):1515–20.
19. Mishra AK, Skrepnik NV, Edwards SG, et al. Efficacy of platelet-rich plasma for chronic tennis elbow: a double-blind, prospective, multicenter, randomized controlled trial of 230 patients. Am J Sports Med 2014;42(2):463–71.
20. Jacobson JA, Chiavaras MM, Lawton JM, et al. Radial collateral ligament of the elbow: sonographic characterization with cadaveric dissection correlation and magnetic resonance arthrography. J Ultrasound Med 2014;33(6):1041–8.

21. Piper SL, Laron D, Manzano G, et al. A comparison of lidocaine, ropivacaine and dexamethasone toxicity on bovine tenocytes in culture. J Bone Joint Surg Br 2012;94(6):856–62.

22. Scherb MB, Han SH, Courneya JP, et al. Effect of bupivacaine on cultured tenocytes. Orthopedics 2009;32(1):26.

23. Finnoff JT, Fowler SP, Lai JK, et al. Treatment of chronic tendinopathy with ultrasound-guided needle tenotomy and platelet-rich plasma injection. PM R 2011;3(10):900–11.

24. Paul T, Braga-Mele R. Bimanual microincisional phacoemulsification: the future of cataract surgery? Curr Opin Ophthalmol 2005;16(1):2–7.

25. Kamineni S, Butterfield T, Sinai A. Percutaneous ultrasonic debridement of tendinopathy-a pilot Achilles rabbit model. J Orthop Surg Res 2015;10:70.

26. Elattrache NS, Morrey BF. Percutaneous ultrasonic tenotomy as a treatment for chronic patellar tendinopathy-jumper's knee. Oper Tech Orthop 2013;23(2): 98–103.

27. Koh JS, Mohan PC, Howe TS, et al. Fasciotomy and surgical tenotomy for recalcitrant lateral elbow tendinopathy: early clinical experience with a novel device for minimally invasive percutaneous microresection. Am J Sports Med 2013;41(3): 636–44.

28. Barnes DE, Beckley JM, Smith J. Percutaneous ultrasonic tenotomy for chronic elbow tendinosis: a prospective study. J Shoulder Elbow Surg 2015;24(1):67–73.

29. Patel MM. A novel treatment for refractory plantar fasciitis. Am J Orthop 2015; 44(3):107–10.

30. Crisp T, Khan F, Padhiar N, et al. High volume ultrasound guided injections at the interface between the patellar tendon and Hoffa's body are effective in chronic patellar tendinopathy: a pilot study. Disabil Rehabil 2008;30(20–22):1625–34.

31. Morton S, Chan O, King J, et al. High volume image-guided injections for patellar tendinopathy: a combined retrospective and prospective case series. Muscles Ligaments Tendons J 2014;4(2):214–9.

32. Maffulli N, Del Buono A, Oliva F, et al. High-volume image-guided injection for recalcitrant patellar tendinopathy in athletes. Clin J Sport Med 2016;26(1):12–6.

33. Chan O, O'Dowd D, Padhiar N, et al. High volume image guided injections in chronic Achilles tendinopathy. Disabil Rehabil 2008;30(20–22):1697–708.

34. Humphrey J, Chan O, Crisp, et al. The short-term effects of high volume image guided injections in resistant non-insertional Achilles tendinopathy. J Sci Med Sport 2010;13(3):295–8.

35. Maffulli N, Spiezia F, Longo UG, et al. High volume image guided injections for the management of chronic tendinopathy of the main body of the Achilles tendon. Phys Ther Sport 2013;14(3):163–7.

36. Alfredson H. Ultrasound and Doppler-guided mini-surgery to treat midportion Achilles tendinosis: results of a large material and a randomised study comparing two scraping techniques. Br J Sports Med 2011;45(5):407–10.

37. Bedi HS, Jowett C, Ristanis S, et al. Plantaris excision and ventral paratendinous scraping for Achilles tendinopathy in an athletic population. Foot Ankle Int 2016; 37(4):386–93.

38. Hall MM, Rajasekaran S. Ultrasound-guided scraping for chronic patellar tendinopathy: a case presentation. PM R 2015. http://dx.doi.org/10.1016/j.pmrj.2015. 10.013.

Past, Present, and Future Considerations for Musculoskeletal Ultrasound

Scott J. Primack, DO

KEYWORDS

- History • Injection • Intervention • Musculoskeletal • Neurologic • Sonography
- Sports • Ultrasound

KEY POINTS

- Musculoskeletal ultrasound has been used since 1958, but its use has increased significantly in recent years.
- Training curricula, certifications, organizational guidelines, and position statements in recent years have helped formalize and standardize the practice of musculoskeletal ultrasound, particularly among nonradiologist musculoskeletal clinicians.
- Future developments in musculoskeletal ultrasound will be fostered by formal ultrasound education programs integrated into residency and fellowship programs.

Confucius stated, "study the past if you would define the future." This clearly holds true for musculoskeletal ultrasound. *Echolocation*, the term used to detect objects and measure distances, was originally developed for nautical purposes. After the sinking of the Titanic, Reginald Fessenden patented the first sonar device capable of detecting an iceberg 2 miles away. By World War I, Paul Langevin and Constantin Chilowsky constructed an underwater sandwich sound generator using quartz and steel plates.[1] The first recorded sinking of a German U-boat using a hydrophone was on April 23, 1916.[2] Between World War I and World War II, ultrasound techniques were used as "reflectoscopes," as a method of detecting flaws or defects in ships and aircraft. The application of echolocation was more widely applied during World War II. These technologies led to the development of the medical diagnostic use of ultrasound.

Ultrasound as a medical diagnostic tool was first used by Dr Karl Dussik in 1942. He attempted to diagnose brain tumors and visualize the cerebral ventricles by measuring transmission of ultrasound beams through the head.[3] The integration of ultrasound into clinical practice was established by Donald and colleagues.[4] He was able to

Disclosures: The author has no commercial or financial conflicts of interest.
Colorado Rehabilitation and Occupational Medicine, 1390 South Potomac Street, Suite 100, Aurora, CO 80012, USA
E-mail address: sprimack@coloradorehab.com

demonstrate the utility of ultrasound in differentiating between cystic and solid abdominal masses.

The first report of musculoskeletal ultrasound was in 1958. Dussik and colleagues[5] was able to describe and measure acoustic attenuation of articular and periarticular tissues. This work led to the first description of anisotropy and the effects of different articular injuries and diseases on ultrasound attenuation, thus laying down the foundation of diagnostic musculoskeletal ultrasound. In 1972, the first B-scan image of a human joint was reported. The clinicians were able to differentiate between a Baker cyst and thrombophlebitis.[6] Just a few years later, Cooperberg and colleagues[7] used ultrasound to demonstrate synovitis in rheumatoid arthritis patients.

With improved technology, musculoskeletal ultrasound began to be increasingly used for detecting shoulder pathology. Crass and colleagues[8] demonstrated the efficacy of ultrasound in the diagnosis of rotator cuff pathology, using surgical correlation as the gold standard. The first outcome-oriented study that used diagnostic ultrasound with a functional outcome measure was done by Harryman and colleagues.[9] Their research demonstrated that a valid functional outcome measure, the Simple Shoulder Test questionnaire, correlated with the integrity of the repaired rotator cuff tendon complex at postsurgical follow-up. The recurrent rotator cuff defect was measured via specific criteria, as described by Mack and colleagues.[10] At the same time, radiologists Fornage[11] and Van Holsbeeck and Introcaso[12] contributed significantly to ultrasound description of the musculoskeletal system.

With advanced engineering in transducers, lower machine cost, and wider availability, there has been a larger trend for nonradiologists to integrate musculoskeletal ultrasound into the clinical assessment. Primack[13] demonstrated that musculoskeletal ultrasound can be used as an extension of the clinical examination. Using ultrasound as the first-line modality for occupational shoulder injuries, it was shown that there was a 40% reduction in imaging cost without compromising quality or accuracy of diagnosis.[14]

Before the twenty-first century, European physicians used sonography as a primary diagnostic tool for neuromusculoskeletal imaging. Martinoli and colleagues[15] were able to describe tendon and nerve sonology. They were able to demonstrate the utility of ultrasound in the detection of loose bodies in joints. One of the challenges of musculoskeletal ultrasound has been that it is operator dependent. Jacobson[16] reviewed that the "non-operator-dependent" quality of MRI is complementary to musculoskeletal sonography. Nazarian[17] pointed out 10 reasons why musculoskeletal ultrasound was an important imaging modality to complement MRI. It has been suggested that MRI is the gold standard for further musculoskeletal ultrasound studies.

By the twenty-first century, musculoskeletal ultrasound was thought efficacious in the musculoskeletal clinician's office. Given the unique ability to visualize soft tissue and bony landmarks accurately, ultrasound has been used for both diagnostic and therapeutic interventions in the outpatient clinical setting with increasing frequency. Given the increasing use of ultrasound as an adjunct in patient management, education has been an ongoing focus for many musculoskeletal clinicians. The American Academy of Physical Medicine and Rehabilitation, American Medical Society for Sports Medicine, American Osteopathic College of Physical Medicine and Rehabilitation, and American Institute of Ultrasound in Medicine, among other organizations, have instituted educational programs to support high demand from clinicians as well as create objectives for competency. A formal musculoskeletal sonography credential was initiated in 2012 by the American Registry for Diagnostic Medical Sonography.

The future is bright in musculoskeletal ultrasound, not only due to advancing technology but also, more importantly, because of the commitment to integrating this imaging modality into resident and fellow education. Coursework objectives have been developed and implemented in the physical medicine and rehabilitation residency program at the Rehabilitation Institute of Chicago since 2008, and other residencies have since followed suit. Finnoff and colleagues[18] proposed a model musculoskeletal course for physical medicine and rehabilitation residents in 2008. In 2015, the American Medical Society for Sports Medicine published a recommended sports ultrasound curriculum for all sports medicine fellowships.[19] The next decade, given the integration of musculoskeletal ultrasound into training curricula, will demonstrate further advances in musculoskeletal ultrasound for both diagnostic uses and therapeutic interventions by educating and training many future leaders in the field.

REFERENCES

1. Hill CR. Medical ultrasonics: an historical review. Br J Radiol 1973;46:899–905.
2. Firestone FA. The supersonic reflectoscope, an instrument of inspecting the interior of solid parts by means of sound waves. J Acoust Soc Am 1945;17:287–99.
3. Dussik KT. On the possibility of using ultrasound waves as a diagnostic aid. Z Neurol Psychiatr 1942;174:153–68.
4. Donald I, MacVicar J, Brown TG. Investigation of abdominal masses by pulsed ultrasound. Lancet 1958;1:1188–95.
5. Dussik KT, Fritch DJ, Kyriazidou M, et al. Measurements of articular tissues with ultrasound. Am J Phys Med 1958;37:160–5.
6. McDonald DG, Leopold GR. Ultrasound B-scanning in the differentiation of Baker's cyst and thrombophlebitis. Br J Radiol 1972;45:729–32.
7. Cooperberg PL, Tsang I, Truelove L, et al. Gray scale ultrasound in the evaluation of rheumatoid arthritis of the knee. Radiology 1978;126:759–63.
8. Crass JR, Craig EV, Thompson RC, et al. Ultrasonography of the rotator cuff: surgical correlation. J Clin Ultrasound 1984;12(8):478–91.
9. Harryman DT II, Mack LA, Wang KY. Repairs of the rotator cuff: correlation of functional results with integrity of the cuff. J Bone Joint Surg Am 1991;73:982.
10. Mack LA, Matsen FA III, Wang KY. Diagnostic ultrasound. St Louis (MO): Mosby; 1991.
11. Fornage BD. Musculoskeletal ultrasound. New York: Churchill Livingstone; 1995.
12. Van Holsbeeck M, Introcaso JH. Musculoskeletal ultrasound. St Louis (MO): Mosby; 1991.
13. Primack SJ. Musculoskeletal ultrasound: the clinician's perspective. Radiol Clin North Am 1999;37:617–21.
14. Primack SJ, Bernton JT, Schauer LM. Diagnostic ultrasound of the shoulder: A cost-effective approach. Presented at the American Academy of Occupational & Evironmental Medicine. Las Vegas, April 28-May 5, 1995.
15. Martinoli C, Bianchi S, Derchi LE. Tendon and nerve sonography. Radiol Clin North Am 1999;37:691–711.
16. Jacobson JA. Musculoskeletal Sonography and M.R. Imaging: a role for both imaging methods. Radiol Clin North Am 1999;37:713–35.
17. Nazarian LN. The top 10 reasons musculoskeletal sonography is an important complementary or alternative technique to MRI. AJR Am J Roentgenol 2008; 190:1621.

18. Finnoff JT, Smith JF, Nutz DJ, et al. A musculoskeletal ultrasound course for physical medicine and rehabilitation residents. Am J Phys Med Rehabil 2010;1(89): 56–69.
19. Finnoff JT, Berkoff D, Brennan F, et al. American Medical Society for Sports Medicine recommended sports ultrasound curriculum for sports medicine fellowships. Clin J Sport Med 2015;25(1):23–9.

Index

Note: Page numbers of article titles are in **boldface** type.

Moving?

Make sure your subscription moves with you!

To notify us of your new address, find your **Clinics Account Number** (located on your mailing label above your name), and contact customer service at:

Email: journalscustomerservice-usa@elsevier.com

800-654-2452 (subscribers in the U.S. & Canada)
314-447-8871 (subscribers outside of the U.S. & Canada)

Fax number: 314-447-8029

Elsevier Health Sciences Division
Subscription Customer Service
3251 Riverport Lane
Maryland Heights, MO 63043

*To ensure uninterrupted delivery of your subscription, please notify us at least 4 weeks in advance of move.

Printed and bound by CPI Group (UK) Ltd, Croydon, CR0 4YY

03/10/2024

01040395-0005